Learning To Love My Cancer

Kay Bevan

Learning To Love My Cancer

How a "silent killer" became a prescription for living

Kay Bevan

with John Bevan, Ed.D.

Charhill Voice, LLC

The people and organizations described herein do not necessarily share views expressed by the authors. Moreover, the brand and product names mentioned herein are trademarks, registered trademarks, or trade names of their respective holders.

First Edition: August, 1999
Printed by: HMS Printing Partnership, Bloomfield, NJ

Cover Design: Raymond Harden
Back Cover Photo: Jo Lackman
Typesetter: Sharon Nicks, *Types*

Publisher's Cataloging-in-Publication
(Provided by Quality Books, Inc.)

Bevan, Kay.
Learning to love my cancer : how a "silent killer" became a prescription for living / by Kay Bevan ; with John Bevan. – 1st ed.
p. cm.
Includes index.
LCCN: 99-93839
ISBN: 0-9671327-0-3

1. Shark cartilage–Therapeutic use. 2. Neovascularization inhibitors–Therapeutic use. 3. Cancer–Alternative treatments. I. Bevan, John (John V.), 1929- II. Title.

RC271.S55B48 1999 616.99'4061
QBI99-616

Library of Congress Catalog Card Number: 99-93839

ISBN Number: 0-9671327-0-3

Published by Charhill Voice, LLC
P.O. Box 344
Sonoita, AZ 85637-0344

Authors' e-mail: char@dakotacom.net
Fax or Phone 520-455-5331

DEDICATION

This book is dedicated to those researchers who ventured outside of toxic pharmaceuticals so that I and others could have a second chance at life.

In the treatment of a sick person, the doctor must be free to use a new therapeutic measure, if in his judgment it offers hope of saving life, re-establishing health, or alleviating suffering.

DECLARATION OF HELSINKI
Adopted by the World Medical Assembly
1964, Helsinki, Finland

(And a guiding principle
of the People Against Cancer, et al.)

"A Voice For The New Millennium"

~

IMPORTANT INFORMATION

This book is for educational and informational purposes only. The reader is encouraged to consult at least one trusted and knowledgeable health care provider before embarking on any dietary or other health-related regimen. The authors and publisher cannot assume responsibility for any adverse effect(s) arising either from the use or misuse of the information contained herein. While an effort was made to provide accurate and useful information for the subject area covered, the authors and publisher assume no responsibility for omissions and errors. Becoming a more informed health care consumer could involve further research and reading as well as seeking out health care professionals for additional opinions and counsel. In any event, the information presented in this book is based largely on one lay person's experience and is in no way intended as a substitute for expert medical counseling and care.

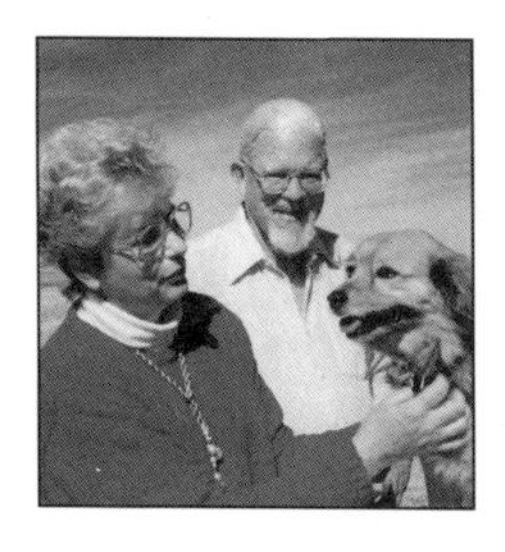

The Authors

Having been married for nearly a half-century, Kay and John Bevan had often worked as a team. Both became public school teachers and were to specialize in adaptive education and thus end their long public careers working with students who had special needs.

While both had attended the Chicago, Illinois public schools, their advanced degrees were earned at the University of Arizona. Kay Bevan received a master's degree in primary/elementary education in 1969 and 13 years later, husband John received a doctor's degree in secondary education with a minor in journalism. Both had also taught school in their respective levels before moving to Tucson, Arizona in 1961. John's work included teaching adult evening classes.

Although it was John who was elected, first, local president, then state president of the American Federation of Teachers in the mid 1960s, it was Kay who was at his side. When Kay became president of the local chapter of the Council for Exceptional Children (CEC) years later, John, who had already served as the chapter's managing editor, stepped in to assist her. Thus, when Kay contracted ovarian/endometrial cancer soon after both had retired from teaching in 1989, they united to fight this implacable disease.

Significantly, both had taught seriously ill children from time to time, but it was John who had worked with numerous students classified as "terminal" and had thus experienced firsthand the frustration, anguish and desperation such a medical prognosis engenders. John received the Arizona CEC "Special Education Teacher of the Year" award in 1980.

Teamed for action yet again, Kay Bevan's chronicle represents quintessential resolve since it was only John who had had some experience in writing. First, he had written commercials for a single radio program followed by limited newspaper work plus, of course, the formal writing associated with his own research and that of academia in general. But of all the projects the two have tackled, this true account is considered the most important. And, actually, both experienced great relief when told its execution actually enhanced its telling.

TABLE OF CONTENTS

Preface

Each of my mornings I greet with enthusiasm feeling grateful that I was able to deny the Specter of Death his morbid wish. Thus each day, whether it be hot or cold, sunny or cloudy, is a shimmering delight. Amazingly, it was a nontoxic "waste" product that made the greatest difference. This is the story of *how* I challenged and beat back the deadly Stage III ovarian/endometrial cancer that had taken over my body.

First, I must issue a caveat: I have never written a book before, not even a short one. I'm a retired primary/elementary school teacher who loves children and animals, sunrises and sunsets and practically everything in between who feels compelled to settle down to some serious business – you. What is imparted here could help save your life.

My husband of 46 years, John, is solidly behind my effort and has suggested – rather, insisted – that his editing was necessary, primarily to ensure brevity. He is a bit of a male chauvinist so I pointed out with some sternness that the subject had to be approached my way. Be aware, however, that any big words or complex sentences are his doing. Remember, I spent 30 years teaching young children.

Kay Bevan
August, 1999

ACKNOWLEDGEMENTS

Since the kindness of scores of people made writing my story possible, I realized any necessary abridgment here would prove difficult if I did not first gratefully note and thank all of those "out there" who assisted me along.

New Jersey cancer researcher, I. William Lane, Ph.D., naturally comes to mind because his pioneering work enabled me to control my cancer and thus to be here in the first place. Curiously, a close neighbor who witnessed my many unexpected turnarounds firsthand, suggested the story should be written. Her name is Shelly Day. She had watched both her mother and brother succumb to this terrible disease of cancer and "knew" I wasn't going to make it.

Then there were still others who also took the time to read the manuscript and offer encouragement and suggestions: Drs. Dante Ruccio, Martin Milner, and Meg Gilbert; Charlotte Christie of The People Against Cancer; Confidant, Marilyn Bollinger; members of Dr. Lane's organization (including Andrew Lane, President of Lane Labs, Inc.; Assistant, David Wales, a driving force behind "getting it done"; Rick Jahnke as well as cancer survivor Marian Murphy); and, interestingly, "typesetter" Sharon Nicks, who, along with graphic artist Raymond Harden, thoughtfully read the manuscript and had taken a personal and kindly interest in the book's completion.

The names of our neighbors who were ever helpful and had graciously included me in their prayers help complete this roster of appreciation: Don and Jo Lackman who had assisted with the photography; Ted and Phyllis Masters; Jim and Midge Cole; Bailey Foster and family; as well as Tom Aylward and his family. All were true neighbors as were the encouraging members of the Patagonia Women's Club.

My own relations, of course, have also been very supportive and happily my paternal aunt, Ann Jepsen, has also been a thriving cancer survivor – and for more than 20 years!

INTRODUCTION

Upon reading the original manuscript of Kay Bevan's deftly written book, I must say excitement took over and I immediately telephoned my colleagues. You see, I am a naturopathic doctor consultant (N.D.C.) and a widely published alternative researcher who had been hoping something like this book would come along. During the course of my ground-breaking but sometimes frustrating work, I refined a nontoxic protocol for the possible control of cancer that had, indeed, saved or prolonged many lives. But sadly, many others were lost because there was no one to take the terminal patient by the hand and actually flesh out the steps necessary to improve one's chance for survival. I told my colleagues that a helping hand now existed in the form of this encouraging and fascinating first person account of survival against incredible odds.

The book's primary heading, *Learning to Love My Cancer*, while perhaps extreme in character and its implied message seemingly improbable, is actually appropriate since the recovered cancer patient must realize the malignancy may remain. But just being able to control the cancer may bring unexpected benefits. For example, the patient may come to view things in a more positive and hopeful light. A living example of this is Kay Bevan, hardly a professional writer, yet sitting down and telling her story with grace and good humor while recalling the futility of her horrible two-year chemotherapy program and the sudden turns in her condition that to this day make her – and others – wonder how she ever made it.

Yet, I do know why, after seven years of living with a very deadly form of cancer, she is alive and well. She had – though almost belatedly – decided on a sensible natural protocol and accepting the help of her husband, John, and the monitoring of some very fine doctors, stayed the course, ignoring any number of dark detractors who crossed her path.

It should be mentioned that while I had heard of the author's experience through the grapevine, I first spoke to her just recently after the book had been mostly written. And unbeknownst to me – and to her, in fact – our experiences regarding this terrible disease were strikingly parallel!

To be sure, I hadn't contracted cancer but Kay Bevan alone had discovered many of the same therapeutic principles and refinements I had in counseling and observing thousands of late-stage cancer patients!

This very personal account of hers is also important because many late-stage cancer victims become paralyzed by the physician's prognosis and even if they do ask probing questions they often confront antipathy for any and all nontoxic therapeutic options. Interestingly, one of the things that the author and her husband discovered early on was that the medical health care industry is truly a business and that there is powerful evidence of a pharmaceutical-medical cartel involving even government bureaucracies and conventional cancer charities.

Even the very recent forays of the giant pharmaceutical companies into the realm of natural medicine must be eyed with suspicion because of a basic conflict of interest. The truly big profits are in selling pharmaceuticals and there may be an interest in stamping out all natural products or to have them reclassified as drugs to insure greater control and profitability. As usual, monetary interest is likely to come before the welfare of the patient. Having long observed this and having retired, I do not charge a consultation fee to any cancer patient who feels a need to call me.

An especially easy read, this book is likewise from the heart and of potential benefit to anyone – from the more casual reader to one in desperate need.

Dr. Dante Ruccio
Newark, New Jersey

chapter one

Innocence

Health had never been an intractable problem for my husband and me although cancer ran in my family. It claimed my father at age 67 as well as his younger sister at 53. Thus on June 17, 1992, when I had a hysterectomy and ovarian cancer was diagnosed, it was not completely unexpected.

Conventional was our outlook toward health matters having sought out M.D.s even for routine eye exams and had never been to a naturopathic physician nor even a chiropractor.

We were married in the Chicago metropolitan area on May 16, 1953. John was 23 years old and myself 19. Teaching beckoned both of us and John soon specialized in adaptive education at the high school level. (I specialized in adaptive education many years later at the primary/elementary level.)

Moving to Tucson, Arizona in 1961, we immediately found new jobs in our respective fields. From the University of Arizona I earned a master's degree and John a doctorate. Professional activities in various organizations captured much of our time and John received the 1980 Teacher of the Year Award from the Arizona Council for Exceptional Children. But in many respects we were an average teaching couple reared in an era of marital stability.

Later, we ventured outside of conventional medicine and came upon treatments that did produce positive results. The move to Tucson greeted us with unexpected pollen allergies. Before an allergy season, some Tucsonans chewed bee wax or cappings daily. We did likewise and it reduced our itching, redness and sneezing markedly.

A worrisome weight problem drove John's weight up to 260 pounds on a 6'1" frame. In 1965 I put him on what was sometimes known as the "Air Force Diet" (later popularized as the Atkins' Diet after Robert C. Atkins, M.D.). He started eating more protein and fewer "junk" carbohydrates and for the first time a diet worked for him. Without the usual hunger and weakness associated with the ordinary calorie diet, his weight dropped to about 230 pounds – a weight level he has maintained to this day.

My chronic rheumatoid arthritis was made much less painful by yet another alternative treatment. Tucson's warm, dry air felt soothing but I started having flare-ups which frequently became incapacitating as the Motrin and Feldene I was taking became less and less effective. Gold therapy suggested by my doctor in 1985 promptly registered: I was in trouble. John came across an old 1972 book written by Giraud W. Campbell, D.O., entitled, *A Doctor's Proven New Home Cure for Arthritis*. My husband briefly skimmed the book and told me the doctor seemed pretty sure of himself. I thought, "A quack, pure and simple," but John prevailed.

The so-called "elimination diet" was a part of Dr. Campbell's regimen which entailed a one-day, water-only fast followed by foods normally considered non-allergenic. Suspect foods are later introduced one at a time. If the ingestion of a particular food is followed the next morning by an arthritic flare-up, you avoid that food for about a week and then try it again. If an untoward reaction reoccurs, you can be reasonably sure it is at least part of the problem. To my surprise, I had such a reaction after eating regular beef. When regular beef was eliminated from my diet, the flare-ups disappeared. Organic beef – beef free of added hormones and antibiotics – did not present a problem. The underlying arthritic pain and inflation remained, but still, the Doctor's regimen helped.

Once again I could spend hours at the malls, window shopping, and John didn't have to carry a lawn chair so that I could sit down every five minutes or so. No longer was the arthritis keeping me home from work. Furthermore, John, who had never thoroughly read a health book in his life, felt quite proud of himself for suggesting that I read the old 1972 book. In 1985 almost all medical doctors said that dietary changes didn't significantly alter the course of arthritis. That's beginning to change now.

The year 1989 brought big changes since we both retired and prepared to move 50 miles southeast of Tucson to a somewhat cooler and beautiful grassland area. Not a town, but rather a "crossroad," Sonoita, Arizona has a windy 5,000-foot elevation and the area is known for its ranches and, lately, its vineyards. It was here in our new country home that I first noticed a strange abdominal pain at the end of November, 1991. My doctor had put me on estrogen-progestogen replacement therapy in 1986 to relieve menopausal symptoms (though it would increase the risk of cancer, I discovered later) and it was thought that the pain may have been related to this treatment. Despite adjustments in the therapy protocol, the pain periodically returned and then worsened until it became unbearable. I was referred to a gynecologist who immediately had me take an ultrasound scan which showed a suspicious cyst on my left ovary. Later, I discovered that a pre-surgery blood test revealed a high CA-125 tumor marker of 118.9, indicating ovarian cancer. Of course, the hysterectomy of June 17, 1992, confirmed it.

Despite our satisfying foray into the alternative realm, we both fell in line when I was diagnosed with the Stage III ovarian/endometrial cancer for even John with his analytic nature saw no other course but the conventional one. The various books I consulted seemed to agree that I faced the battle of my life and the likelihood of winning was dim.

On the other hand, John tended to ignore my foreboding partly out of habit and partly because the oncologist and his office staff seemed so upbeat. Besides, the lab reported that most of the cancer cells were well-differentiated and thus less aggressive. We thought the following: any research breakthroughs would be promulgated immediately; if there was a promising treatment "out there", my oncologist would know about it; everyone was interested in the control of cancer or its cure and surely the pharmaceutical companies were doing everything possible to save lives and would not let self-interest stand in the way of a nontoxic, relatively inexpensive treatment. You see why this chapter is entitled, "Innocence."

chapter two

One, Two, Three and You're...

Chemotherapy poisons the body to kill cancer cells. About as many normal cells are damaged or killed as malignant ones. The less effective chemicals of the past often killed patients. This is not to say patients no longer die from chemotherapy. They do. The hardest hit are the fast growing cells which often include the malignant ones. But the normal cells found in hair follicles and linings of the gastrointestinal tract, for example, also are fast growers. This is why one undergoing chemotherapy often experiences hair loss and digestive upsets. The body's rebellion is its way of telling you something, as Providence intended. John and I knew this. Still, I had high hopes. Even John's hard questioning of the oncologist didn't dim my optimism. Albeit noncommittal, my oncologist seemed hopeful.

Carboplatin came first. The course started July 2, 1992, and was to consist of six IV doses. The third treatment was delayed one week because of a low white blood platelet count. But that seemed inconsequential since each treatment was spaced three weeks apart anyway and – surprise – I was feeling fine! Even up to and past the fifth treatment, I had no nausea, no great loss of appetite, no hair loss. True, I was taking another chemical, Torecan, to curb nausea, but I was shopping, running errands, doing everything I normally did. Some loss of energy was the only symptom of the poison coursing through my body. Even the nurses seemed astonished and some predicted that I might have an easier time than most.

But this was not to be as I developed an uneasy feeling and a pain surfaced behind my left knee. The pain took on a character unlike that of my arthritis. I applied hot compresses, cold compresses, took Tylenol, but nothing helped. The leg became swollen but not warm to the touch. The pain increased. My oncologist seemed deeply concerned when I finally telephoned him. "Be careful. Don't squeeze it, don't bend it, keep it straight out," he said. "It may be a blood clot and we don't want it to break free." He ordered me to come to the hospital the following morning and to bring my hospital bag. An ultrasound scan revealed a clot and I was hospitalized for anticoagulant treatments given through yet another IV. For five days my blood was drawn every six hours to measure its coagulation time and slowly I was weaned from the drug Heparin to Coumadin. I remained on this "blood thinner," Coumadin, some four months following the hospital stay.

A short time later, April 20, 1993, a laparoscopic probe of the abdominal cavity revealed miniscule outcroppings. The tiny tumors remained very much an unwanted guest. But the surgeon (who is my oncologist) emphasized to my husband just how tiny the specks were. Nevertheless, the fact that he had inserted a Port-a-Cath, its tube winding into my abdomen in preparation for the powerful Mitoxantrone to be drained directly into the cavity, clearly revealed what lay ahead.

* * * *

During all of these hospital stays, my husband visited me every day often announcing, "Pup and I have everything under control." (The name of our little poodle/spaniel mix is actually "Coco.") He would give an account of all the things he did to keep the house in tiptop shape say, from taking out the garbage, to vacuuming the walk areas (never the corners) to not using the dishes so they wouldn't stack up. Boiling water to heat sausages was the extent of his cooking. Otherwise, he ate cold food and used paper towels for plates.

His bragging notwithstanding, it became apparent that he was not able to take care of himself. He had little experience in doing traditional "women's work" and it all was quite a challenge. He reported that our dog kept looking for me. I wondered why?

The nurses, in the meantime, were having difficulty inserting IV needles – and no wonder! Having had so many insertions, the veins were in full rebellion bubbling up and then collapsing and at times there would be three nurses around me trying different places on my hands and arms. Once it took them 40 minutes! My body was telling me something but I wasn't listening. But, alas, this problem was not to be the worst of my experiences.

* * * *

Backing up some I should mention that the sixth scheduled treatment of Carboplatin had been canceled because of the blood clot. For the first time I was suffering some inconvenience. For a short time, shopping or just moving about required the use of a wheelchair to keep my leg in an horizontal position.

I should also mention that just before I was diagnosed with cancer, John splurged and bought a new 1992 Lincoln Town Car. Being frugal, John's purchase of this behemoth I called "a living room on wheels" was unexpected. But surprisingly, it proved especially useful as he could adjust the front passenger seat forward so that I was able to stretch out in back and position my left leg properly. Since living in a rural area required considerable driving, its size and smooth ride proved a definite plus.

It wasn't long until I was walking again only having to wear elastic stockings to help prevent embolisms.

Before the second course of chemotherapy was to begin, excitement filled the air as my oncologist tried to get me into an experimental treatment program he was involved with. It promised to be less toxic because proteins which had an affinity to malignant cells were attached to radioactive agents. Theoretically, a higher percentage of the normal cells would be spared. However, my case didn't meet the established protocol and unhappily I was turned down. (Many months later, I was to learn that the clinical trial didn't turn out as hoped. Apparently, the proteins and radioactive agents separated.)

The second course, consisting of six scheduled intraperitoneal chemotherapy sessions, began June 1, 1993, and my reaction to it was immediate. Mitoxantrone was drained into the abdominal cavity via the Port-a-Cath. Each treatment lasted two or three hours. Another agent was introduced through an IV to help lessen any side effects. Besides the frustration involved in having the poor nurses struggle to insert an IV needle, the abdominal pain, bloating, nausea, vomiting and retching that did follow a treatment was especially severe and early on the interval between treatments was increased from three weeks to four. In fact, my oncologist who initially had expressed high hopes for this procedure now considered stopping it. But I said that if the chemical holds hope of killing off the cancer, let's continue.

While all of this was happening, the pain behind my left knee resurfaced July 8, 1993, but, thankfully, an ultrasound scan showed no clot. Besides the periodic blood test to gauge the white cell count already mentioned, imaging was done from time to time to check for possible blood clots and tumor metastases.

The severe pain and discomfort continued even during intervals when it was expected to diminish so on December 7 an upper and lower barium scan was ordered to check for adhesions and any blockages. My digestive system was "unobstructed" and with just a hint of a shrug I was told it was simply the side effects of the chemotherapy. Haplessly, I now developed a hiatal hernia and had to sleep with my head elevated.

On October 6, my second course of six abdominal infusions had come to an end and thus when I developed a retching episode on December 13 it was alarming. I had grown weak from chronic digestive problems and constipation and now I was retching hour after hour and I couldn't stop. John half carried me to the car and we rushed to the emergency room once again. There, flat x-rays showed an intestinal blockage. Barium was found left over from the scan that was done several days before! Medicine was administered to reduce the spasms and I had to go on a clear liquid diet to help dissolve the solidified barium.

In January of 1994, 1 had to select a new primary care physician from my HMO's list. I had joined the HMO through my school system in 1988. It was a not-for-profit organization with a good reputation. By discreetly asking questions of several nurses and by talking to patients, I gathered enough information to make my decision. Picking this particular doctor for my primary care turned out to be a critically fortunate move as you will see later.

In February, I was feeling somewhat better but still losing weight. In one week I had lost four pounds. Altogether, I lost about 30 pounds since being diagnosed with cancer. One relief, the abdominal Port-a-Cath was removed.

March saw the side effects continue intermittently and despite a return to the emergency room to again curb out-of-control retching, there was, overall, some improvement. This last retching episode, though, did have one unique feature, I couldn't even keep an ounce of water down.

The week of April 4 was important as I underwent preparation for an onocostint scan. The injection of a radioactive substance which only locked onto malignant cells produced "lights" on an x-ray plate. The film of my abdominal cavity had many of these, including an hourglass cluster on the left side. The little devils were still with me and I braced for yet another round.

* * * *

The summer of 1994 was pivotal despite my dim prospects. Having always registered but little interest in health matters, John swung around 180 degrees to confront my peril, sometimes cussing some in the process. His help was welcomed, but still, what an unlikely source for health advice!

Thankfully, the third course of chemotherapy hadn't been that bad. It was Mitomycin-C with 5-fluorouracil (5-FU) also taken through a series of six IV's (needle insertion was still very difficult). However, the CA-125 markers that had held steady for nearly two years started an ominous rise.

This marker measures the concentration of certain blood proteins which tends to correspond to the seriousness of certain cancers – especially ovarian. An elevated marker signals advanced cancer growth. Any marker at or below 35 is considered in the "safe" range. While it can be thrown off by other physical conditions and is otherwise not always perfectly accurate, it still remains the premier gauge of ovarian cancer. The May 19, 1994, marker had risen to 28.5 from the 7.3 of two months earlier and things were not looking up.

This is when John began to stir and he thought there might be an experimental treatment "out there" that could be of some help. His voice didn't ring solidly but he dug in and we toured the local libraries and book stores. We purchased a bundle of books including, *Sharks Don't Get Cancer* by I. William Lane, Ph.D., and Linda Comac. Somehow, this of all books was misplaced and forgotten.

About a year or so earlier, February 28,1993, the shark cartilage study of Cuba was featured on "60 Minutes." The segment followed 29 terminal cancer patients in a hospital-controlled clinical trial. Reportedly, CBS Television had spent $350,000 to make sure the study was legitimate. But we were still so focused on the conventional, we paid the segment no heed. Unfortunately, we missed the July, 1993, repeat and update. (At this time about half had survived and were getting better.) Nevertheless, John uncovered Dr. Lane's book which featured the Cuban study and asked if I had read it. I had not. He took a deep breath, sat down and hunched over it. Reading with unusual intensity, he quickly finished it. His bearing told the story, shark cartilage was in my future. "I think there is something to it," were his exact words. After reading the book myself, I agreed, but I must admit that by this time hope not only failed to "spring eternal," it hardly beckoned. The painful abdominal pressure I had felt before being diagnosed was coming back.

The third and last course of chemotherapy ended June 8, 1994, with a whimper. The tumor marker of June 24 registered, 130.1 and six days later we were back in the oncologist's office. Obviously frustrated, my oncologist said the three courses of chemo hadn't done much good and for now it would have to be the gentler hormonal therapy. Casually, I mentioned trying to bolster my immune system in a variety of ways including the taking of vitamins and minerals. He, too, took supplements as a precaution and generally seemed favorably disposed toward my efforts. However, John had just read an article about the favorable outcome of the Cuban shark cartilage study and when he started questioning the oncologist about it, the doctor's demeanor changed.

The oncologist was trying to write out a prescription for Tamoxifen, one of the hormonal agents, while John was asking such questions as: Are Cuban doctors well trained? Has the Cuban study been reported on in any of the medical journals? And so on. The oncologist was seemingly upset by this line of inquiry and he continually made errors in trying to write out the prescription. When the doctor pulled out another prescription pad, John finally stopped his questioning and a prescription form was then completed.

At that point the nurse came in and took us aside. After some quiet conversation, she told us that this gentler hormonal therapy would have to do because my immune system "couldn't be pounded anymore." It would be Tamoxifen alternated with Megace (Megestrol). And, thus, it was just two years into my conventional treatment, June 30, 1994, that we were told that my case was essentially terminal and the only realistic hope was to slow the cancer down.

I could now sympathize with my oncologist whom I had grown to like, for now I was rattled. But strangely, John was still calm.

chapter three

No... No... Not the Chemo!

The gravity of my case did not immediately penetrate John's awareness. Within hours, however, he erupted into a whirl of sound and motion. He must have wanted to keep me because never before had I observed such fury and focus. Always questions! He targeted anyone who might know something, especially about shark cartilage. We thought its promise was too good to be true and were fighting off waves of darkness and doubt so that we might keep an open mind and come to a definitive conclusion – yes or no – as to whether it realistically might spare my life. We were in and out of health food stores, pharmacies, libraries, book stores, the homes of "health nuts." But especially, John was on the phone. In fact, he became hoarse.

He did telephone a local distributor of health products whose husband had colon cancer and ended up in a hospice with only two months to live. She had begun giving him some 15 grams of shark cartilage daily in capsule form and she said that he lived several months longer than expected, but this was hardly conclusive evidence of cartilage efficacy. The daily dosage she administered was too little and the brand chosen was not specifically processed for the possible control of cancer – and it was strike one. She knew less about shark cartilage than John did.

Later, John somehow received a telephone call from the office of a retirement community and the manager or someone in the office volunteered that several men there had tried shark cartilage, "and it didn't do them a bit of good." Again the questions: What kind of cancer did they have? Liver and prostate was the reply. Do you know what brand they used? He didn't. Did they take the capsule or powder form? Capsule, he thought. Is it possible to talk to them? No, they died. How long were they on the cartilage before they died? "Oh-h-h one was on it a week and a half and the longest perhaps a month and a half." Strike two. Because these men had too little time remaining for the slow-acting cartilage to do any good, there was nothing conclusive in this part of town.

In fact, John found nothing conclusive anywhere he investigated. John had bypassed those with a financial interest in the sale of shark cartilage products and, resultingly, he could not uncover a single case in which cartilage saved a life. What did John finally conclude? There was, indeed, something to the cartilage therapy after all!

* * * *

You need to know up front, John is a little crazy. I guess I tend to be a little hard on him thus be assured his craziness is not all bad, just confounding. Let me try to explain by going back some.

In the mid 1960's, John decided, out of the blue, to decorate our newly purchased Tucson home which had a hint of Spanish styling, many warm nooks, and was built around its curved lot. Its purchase was my choice. Never had he taken an interest in color coordination (God, no!), nor decorating, nor architecture. But now he took charge! He had deep red carpeting laid in the living areas. He brought in rough-hewned Spanish wooden furniture he found on sale and his eyes locked onto a huge iron *outdoor* Spanish wall lantern to put up in the living room! The store's proprietor felt my embarrassment. This thing measured some 30 inches high and 18 inches wide and it was dull black with many rust accents (i.e. just plain rust). But John wouldn't be dissuaded and it took center stage inside, next to the front door. A huge candle went into the center holder. "Good light in the event of a power outage," John concluded.

Neighbors came over, their eyes and mouths held wide, and invariably asked who did the decorating. I had to point to John. The resulting decor was odd, but beautiful! Even the furniture store's proprietor made a special trip to look at it and pronounced it, "Interesting."

John committed one big boo-boo, however. He painted the walls of the main bedroom a pumpkin color and then had pumpkin color carpeting laid. Whew! Talk about clash. He wasn't about to repaint the walls so hc pondered his blunder and came up with a startling solution. Select some red furniture, red drapes, and red bed covering and "it should all come together in beautiful harmony." And unbelievably it worked!

A decade later, John decided a six-foot-high wall across the middle of our front yard would create a nice patio. He finally found a contractor willing to erect it and I must say the neighbors were wary. The front of the pie-shaped lot was well over 100 feet across and this newly created private area was considerable. The wall curved so that it appeared to be an extension of the house. With its classic detailing, it was strikingly beautiful! For weeks people stopped in front and once again I had to point to John, this time as the architect!

His reputation thus enhanced, our neighbors across the way were inspired to build a mother-in-law dwelling behind their house but the wife complained its front yard also would serve as back yard of the main house. John moseyed over, surveyed the scene thoughtfully – perhaps a full 10 seconds – and suggested turning the planned house some 70 or 80 degrees so each would have its own front and rear area. It was done and what an improvement!

The question may arise, other people were heeding him, so why don't I listen? Well, I do, sort of...

* * * *

One must remember my chance for long-term survival was close to zero. It was truly dark outside. The recent expressions of my oncologist and his nurse weren't the only indicators. This prognosis was part of every medical book I had read. "Oh, just stop reading!" suggested the smiling oncology nurse. I didn't stop reading, but I was listening to John more than I ever had. Indeed, desperation prevailed.

At times the uncertainty we felt crippled our resolve to forge ahead because this feeling was so pervasive and wearing. Having done some research in education, John knew that research could be rigged to favor a predetermined outcome and that this was more common than most people suspected. He distrusted testimonials not that they were wholly useless, but because even sincere people often draw unreliable conclusions.

Even ever-present fortuity contributed its ragged edge to the strain. We happened to watch the first "60 Minute" segment on the Cuban shark cartilage study but missed the follow-up repeat. We came close to not buying the book, *Sharks Don't Get Cancer* and then misplaced it. Conceivably, it could have gathered dust for months and not just a week or so. Had we come across reading materials that disparaged cartilage therapy in these early days or had my oncologist said something negative, we might not have pursued it. My oncologist – bless him – did us a big favor by saying, "I don't know" to almost all of John's questions. He said that it was impossible to keep up with all the medical research out there. We were to talk to M.D.s who would express loose opinions as hard fact. In fact, we came to know few who would admit to not knowing. It was obvious that we were essentially on our own and that we would have to choose our course based on the information available. We found the information in Dr. Lane's book, *Sharks Don't Get Cancer*, most helpful.

* * * *

A state licensed naturopathic physician (N.M.D or N.D.) had recently started her practice in the nearby town of Patagonia. At my behest, John called her to make an appointment and to briefly discuss my taking shark cartilage. She had heard no reports of toxicity and suggested safety was not an issue. Thus, very tentatively, I prepared to take it. John volunteered to drink some of the powder mixed in a glass of tomato juice to see if he had a bad reaction to it. He had none. "But it tastes God-awful," he said. (No flavored powder was then available).

The big day was July 12, 1994. Taste being the least of my worries, on this date I started ingesting it orally, rapidly increasing the daily allotment from about 20 grams to 60 grams taken in four separate doses spread throughout the day to effect systemic saturation. Very soon after, I started taking two of the four daily doses by retention enema. John felt more comfortable with this compromise since the subjects of the Cuban study used only retention enemas for the first six weeks. But interestingly, most participants opted to continue the retention enemas after this six-week period even though given the choice of taking the cartilage powder orally. Nevertheless, further experience was demonstrating that taking the cartilage powder orally (on an empty stomach and well before a meal) was effective.

Each oral dose consisted of about 15 grams of the powder thoroughly mixed with about seven ounces of low sodium V-8 juice or some other recommended liquid and was taken on an empty stomach usually about one half-hour (now, one full hour) before eating to get it past the stomach acids quickly. (In fact, some people, I learned, took 1/8 teaspoon of bicarbonate of soda with a little water about 10 minutes before drinking the cartilage/liquid mixture to neutralize the stomach acids a bit.) This procedure should increase the bioavailabilty of the macro proteins believed to be the key active ingredients of the cartilage. Each dosage was made fresh each time. It is thought that the cartilage cuts off the blood supply to the tumor (antiangiogenesis), starving it of nutrients needed to grow or maintain itself. Needless to say, it is thus more likely to be effective against solid tumors than non-solid cancers such as leukemia.

For each of the two retention enemas, I poured the water/ powder mixture into a clean plastic Fleet brand enema container (the original contents were first emptied). I used about four ounces of tepid water (body temperature) and mixed it very thoroughly with the shark cartilage powder. This Fleet container seemed to work better than the standard apparatus and lasted for about a month. Talk about recycling! The enema dosages were also mixed fresh each time.

Not surprisingly, when the time did come to do the retention enemas, I felt some hesitancy as it involved retaining the mixture for at least 30 minutes. But soon, I was often able to retain them indefinitely! Unlike a regular enema that cleanses the colon, the retention enema, as the term implies, results in the colonic absorption of the cartilage mixture into the blood stream. Lying on the right side for at least the initial minutes was the procedure I used.

To be sure, I did experience a few "accidents" (for which I was prepared), but only at the beginning. Surprisingly, it became a restful time as I usually listened to the radio. It should be emphasized that I always used clinical grade shark cartilage – now, the BeneFin brand.

The taking of at least one gram of the cartilage daily for every two pounds of body weight is critical: a 100-pound person would thus take <u>at least</u> 50 grams of the cartilage daily. To speed up antiangiogenesis and thus recovery, I sometimes took 95 or even 115 grams of the cartilage per day in at least five or six dosages, some taken at night to spread it out. Since I weighed roughly 125 pounds at these times, the ratio amounted to nearly one gram of cartilage to one pound of body weight. It is disheartening to hear of people taking the *small* dosages listed on the cartilage container for ordinary dietary supplementation, having drawn the conclusion that this low dosage level is appropriate for the control of cancer. Government regulations disallow a more complete guide on the container itself!! **For this and other reasons, it is my**

belief one should always consult a knowledgeable health care professional as we did before embarking on such a program.

The naturopathic physician spoken of earlier turned out to be remarkably patient and she did a superb job assisting us through the uncharted waters that loomed so troublingly ahead. Besides sanctioning the shark cartilage therapy, she suggested a Hoxsey-like formula which is similar to another herbal mixture called Essiac. (It is interesting to note that the two formulas were developed many miles apart and the developers of each were unknown to one another). Other herbs and enzymes on her recommended list also became a part of my arsenal.

Informative rather than directive, this naturopathic physician provided us with an interactive experience. She noted that taking at least some of the cartilage by retention enema was especially appropriate for me as I was still experiencing gastrointestinal upsets caused by past chemotherapy. "The terminally ill patients in the Cuban study no doubt took it that way partly for the same reason," she said.

We noticed that she was forced to charge an eight percent sales tax on the natural medicines she prescribed. This struck us as odd since in Arizona there is no state tax on prescribed pharmaceuticals nor even on food (except when eaten inside restaurants or fast food places). She noted that the wealthiest segment of the pharmaceutical industry has such a tight grip on health care that anything or anybody that might conceivably compete with it is placed at a disadvantage. Because politicians often respond to the pharmaceutical industry's monetary clout, many natural medicinal products are taxed, she suggested. Clearly, though, this regressive tax hurts the poor in general and some terminal cancer patients in particular.

* * * *

This juncture seems appropriate to test John's reasoning as to why I am now depending on sharks and some back-up substances many people would label nostrums or elixirs. You be the judge.

John had noticed that terminally ill persons thrown out on their own typically become totally confused as to what to do (as was I). They had been inculcated with the notion that the "toxic" approach with its fast response time was the ideal (true of both of us) . Often they knew of no knowledgeable person to consult when told, "All has failed" and in grasping at straws they were tentative and used the pharmaceutical model in making their critical decisions. (Thus, those who grasped at the shark cartilage approach had no concept of the slower speed involved in using a natural, low-tech product nor were they aware of the greater dosages likely to be required.) They would wait until signs of imminent death surfaced and then act when it was hopelessly late. Then, as per the pharmaceutical paradigm, they would follow the dosages on the container – the only ones allowed by bureaucratic edict – which would seem entirely reasonable to them and they would thus ingest far too little of it to be effective. And, invariably, they would die as their M.D.s had predicted. According to John we are talking here about doing harm for profit a la the tobacco industry.

Then why is it that he trusts Dr. I. William Lane, the cartilage guru? Well, he doesn't. John is one of those beings who tends to trust no one, not even himself as will soon be evident. On top of all this, since John seems a little crazy, I also question him. I'm beginning to wonder, though, if the proverbial "method" of his might not be madness after all?

Enough said. For better or worse, my loving husband and I were embarked on a voyage of hope and discovery on a sea filled with sharks – sharks of all kinds!

chapter four

In the Beginning...

About one week into the cartilage therapy, my long-standing rheumatoid arthritis symptoms unexpectedly faded away. To be sure, this side benefit of the cartilage therapy (along with its potential to ease psoriatic skin disease) was known to us. But these arthritis symptoms had tended to lurk well behind my concern over the ovarian cancer which, of course, had taken center stage.

Trying to describe the gnawing pain, swelling and stiffness of arthritis to someone who has never had the disease, is difficult. While hardly ever fatal, it can have devastating consequences. It was a happy day when I discovered that the dietary change already mentioned curbed the more serious flare-ups. Still, my knuckles were swollen rather grotesquely, requiring the re-sizing of my rings. Although I was able to function, it was draining, not only physically, but mentally as well. It was as though my body was harnessed by a ball and chain and had a fiery devil taking jabs at every joint and then mocking every move with still more pain.

A good night's sleep was an infrequent luxury. Sometimes the early morning alarm brought some relief because the night had been spent in suspended wakefulness. But the waking hours to follow, bled by chronic exhaustion, bore its own class of tedium.

At times the pain just stuck. It was this unrelentingness that made me most want to find agents promising real relief. What a surprise to find that such agents would not be the aspirin, nor Zostrix, not even Motrine nor Feldene, all classic agents of the medical establishment, but a simple dietary change and now, incredibly, a lowly waste product, shark cartilage. And following the start of my cartilage therapy, the symptoms vanished!

John and I refused to celebrate this unexpected outcome as we knew it didn't necessarily mean I would have similar success in controlling my cancer. Besides, an abdominal pressure had been edging into my consciousness for some weeks now and though not very painful, it was similar to the pressure I felt before my cancer diagnosis.

* * * *

It was John's thinking that strict regimentation would enhance my prospects in challenging the malignancy. He thus established himself as my outrider and I couldn't get away with anything! If I wanted to scrub a day's quota of cartilage because of fatigue or gastrointestinal distress, he made sure I didn't. Even the naturopathic physician seemed to approve of his support and active interest in making sure I followed a strict regimen. True, I had promised to "honor and obey" him back in '53 but now his chauvinistic attitude was no longer that humorous.

Everything had a timetable. If we had to be out somewhere, all my mixing apparatus came along so that I could ingest the powder/juice mix at precisely the appointed times. He did suggest taking the capsules when away and it did make it somewhat easier, but I was taking such large dosages that it was rather impractical. Besides, it was thus more expensive.

If for some reason oral ingestion became impossible, a retention enema was substituted. He checked everything precisely. A few times he used our gram scale to check the cartilage containers for weight consistency! (They varied very little). He double checked mathematically my daily allotment average. If, for example, I was actually averaging 65 grams daily, a pound container should last very close to seven days. And if it didn't I was alerted. Not only did he keep an account of every dosage, but also of any symptoms he thought significant.

He approached my course of treatment much the same way

he had explored interior decorating and architectural projects, with consummate energy and focus. Only this time, of course, the outcome wasn't likely to be just a clash of colors if all fails. We both realized, too, that uncertainty was going to be a constant companion regardless of any "proofs" of cartilage efficacy that might emerge along the way.

The reason John gave for his fastidiousness is interesting: A strict protocol exercised around-the-clock by highly knowledgeable nurses and doctors is de riqueur in a hospital-controlled clinical trial. To John, this appeared to be the reason the Cuban shark cartilage study over time had such a positive outcome. On the contrary, for the reasons already suggested, only a small percentage of terminal patients taking cartilage on their own succeed in saving themselves. In a nutshell, it amounted to a lack of knowledge and discipline. And my case – whether one likes to view it this way or not – is a clinical trial involving just one subject, me.

* * * *

Absolute was the loneliness and isolation I felt as I trembled before that which stretched so far and beyond. My appearance was such, that many people seemed to reflect my dismal prospects by their comments and stabs at hopefulness. But I wasn't likely to be around for long so why should people get too close or even talk of my having a future? After all, my own perspective was limited to the next special event – say, the next birthday, anniversary, holiday or even the next doctor visit. At this time in mid 1994, I was looking only as far as my husband's birthday, November 12.

Often, I would just hug the nurses, my doctor and even my husband who despite appearances is actually very huggable and cuddly. (How he fought this revelation!) Even our little dog was receiving my special attention as she had proven such a faithful and warm companion.

(John thinks portions of what I have narrated so far –

including some of the longer segments about him – are hardly relevant, but I disagree. One has to experience the uncertainty of cancer to understand why. I've come to the conclusion that my story resides largely in the details of my thoughts and feelings and not simply in sparse sketches. So I told him to bug out.)

An encouraging tumble of my tumor marker from 130.1 of June 24, 1994, to 97.8 six weeks later was yet another turn happily received. Impulsively, we allowed for the possibility that the cartilage was responsible, but I had only been on it for three weeks! Ordinarily, 12 to 24 weeks of therapy were required for such an improved marker change.

But it was just several weeks later, August 28, that the painful abdominal pressure that had been dogging me now for two or three months suddenly eased and then disappeared. This event occurred about seven weeks into my cartilage therapy, just about the time one should expect based on clinical experience.

Thus encouraged by the responses, John spoke of our experiences to a coworker whose wife also had terminal cancer, but was so close to death the cartilage hardly had any chance of working in time. And it didn't. Although this young woman was not well known to us, I truly felt the pain of her death and wondered of the outcome had this therapy been available for her some months earlier.

It was during this time we were accumulating a library of health books and journals and even audio and video tapes as John's investigatory instincts exploded into virtually all facets of the health field. And conversant in health matters he became.

Previously, John had no interest in health matters and keeping tabs of our health needs had been relegated to my sphere. When he finally did stir, his very first conclusion was, "There is no war against cancer." And he had questions about the $30 billion funneled into it. This conclusion appeared to come out of the blue and since the vestigial effects of the chemotherapy had me in its grip I had no strength to explore his line of information and reasoning. God knows where such an exchange would have led anyway. Back when he popped his unexpected "expertise" in architecture and interior decorating, there appeared to be no link between his educational background, nor even past interest, with the beatific result. The conclusion I reached then? The aesthetic outcome was an accident, though a happy one.

* * * *

Since the February 28, 1993, "60 Minutes" program was pivotal to my starting on the shark cartilage treatment, John telephoned CBS in New York and tried to order a video of the complete follow-up program aired in July. His interest was not only in our watching the original segment but also the circumferential commentary of the July repeat we had missed. But he was only able to order a video of the shark cartilage segment itself. Upon seeing the segment again, however, we were amazed at the tricks the mind can play.

Our impression after the viewing it back in 1993 was that cartilage therapy was, essentially, without foundation, a desperate experimental reach in the war against cancer. The positive impressions of the study instead came from our reading reports of an outcome one would not expect: a nearly 50 percent survival rate plus reports of autopsy x-rays showing that five of the subjects who did die had tumors in clear dissolution (Swiss cheese appearance) as well as having learned that others investigating the study had also found it promising.

And how transformed our impression became after watching the segment again many months later. Possessed of newly acquired insights honed by our frantic exploration of health issues, the study participants seemed now to be each juggling a hot potato. The producers of the segment were "skeptical"; the trenchant Mike Wallace appeared guarded and his opening exchange with Cuba's lead medical specialist, by centering on the skepticism to which the doctor might be subjected, heightened the apprehension.

Three highly placed oncology specialists, including two NCI-trained Americans, examined the patients and/or their x-rays and other records and each found evidence of some tumor regression. Each one seemed uncomfortable, but the last U.S. specialist consulted appeared especially so. He was asked by the producers to examine the patient x-rays without being apprised of the protocol agent. After two hours of concentration, he concluded, "there is some regression to follow up on." And Mike Wallace then revealed the agent, shark cartilage. Was the doctor familiar with it? "No-o-o-o" said he, a disbelieving lilt suggesting more than just surprise.

Some suggest that immediately following a surprise event, those involved tend to be the most forthright to the point of even going counter to their perceived self-interest. This may be the reason why auto insurance companies suggest that their policy holders say little immediately following an accident. It has been my experience that those who are suddenly forced to come to a troubling conclusion, over time shift it to a more comfortable alignment with their self-interest. It goes without saying, the same phenomenon may be observed in the health care industry. Two examples follow:

One early researcher who had uncovered the antiangiogenic potential of shark cartilage, objected to his name being used by the Cuban study's lead promoter, Dr. Lane, even though the work had been long published!

A second early researcher at the Institut Jules Bordot – "the Sloan-Kettering of Western Europe," concluded Lane – resisted publishing his animal studies saying that the results were not significant. But a U.S. research analyst carefully studied the Belgian data and, indeed, they showed shark cartilage repressed tumor growth in five of the nine experiments!

The term "montebank" was used as part of a question directed to Dr. Lane apparently because he stood to profit from his research work despite the fact that one seldom finds a researcher (or journalist for that matter) working for nothing.

Cancer patients were warned that taking shark cartilage on their own could get them into trouble and were sternly counseled to undergo a full complement of the toxic therapies before even considering cartilage. Only if all else failed was such a therapy to be considered. This is the course I followed and little did I know that the vomiting, the retching, the weight loss and the pain from my chemotherapy would have a legacy undreamed of!

In all, thc negative overlay filtered out many of the therapy's legitimate rays of promise and upon seeing the segment initially we simply saw no reason to respond to it.

Medical "experts" still suggest that nothing significant was accomplished by the Cuban study because it was done outside the formal peer review structure. If two U.S. oncology specialists trained in the research methodology of the National Cancer Institute does not constitute peer review, what does? One should note that other physicians and experienced observers were also there.

Others suggest that the producers of the "60 Minutes" program were duped, that the study at best was weak. But careful analyses seems to suggest the opposite. One of the observations made by the first U.S. cancer specialist was that many of the patients in the study were too far gone and shouldn't have been included in the first place. This automatically skews the outcome in such a way as to conceal its strength. It obviously wasn't rigged to bring about a favorable outcome. How often do montebanks go out seeking the inspection of outsiders? You may want to answer that question yourself.

* * * *

Because my life is in the balance, John and I have a vested interest in coming as close to the truth as possible. For you to review the facts of my case and to factor them in with whatever else appears appropriate may be the prudent course. But the informational milieu is such a chaotic tangle that truly one needs a scalpel to cut through it all. And I must warn, the task is daunting. But if people with terminal diseases somehow find alternative cures or controls, this may illuminate paths for others. Trying and failing is one thing. Not trying is something else.

One might hear an expert concluding – and with quite an air, in fact – that a personal account such as mine is worthless because it is "anecdotal." Somewhat in his defense, it must be said that a true cause-and-effect relationship is not always easy to establish. Then there are the true believers, people who seldom can be believed. Apparently in need of certainty, they sometimes imagine a life threatening disease, find an exotic treatment and report a marvelous cure. John says they are easy to spot because of the air of absolute certainty they exude in their pronouncements. No fear have they!

When you visit an M.D. and he prescribes something, he may say, "We'll try this and see if it clears up your condition." To him this is a legitimate investigatory approach as long as the agent is a pharmaceutical or something else in the conventional inventory. Typically, however, an inexpensive natural product, even one with a long history of positive service, given in the same way by an outside practitioner and with beneficent results, is still relegated to the anecdotal domain!

As a class, patient testimonials must be suspect. But there are those that are compelling. We had a friend who suffered a "nervous stomach" even when calm and relaxed. Overproduction of stomach acid was thought to be the cause and a thorough physical examination bore this out. It proved to be chronic and more severe than average. Because it wasn't that serious, high dosages of a conventional antacid was recommended. And because he suffered much less when taking the high dosages, it was considered effective by both him and the doctor. This conclusion was also validated whenever he forgot to take it as his symptoms again emerged; and when he lowered the dosage, the symptoms made a partial return. Now, one could suggest other events were intervening, but if this probable cause-and-effect relationship remained unchallenged over time, the conclusion becomes all the more obvious. This, of course, is an anecdotal account few would seriously argue about. Still, he may have been influenced by the doctor suggesting that it would work and all or part of the positive outcome thus stemmed from the mind/body connection. Significantly, placebo-controlled experiments while showing such responses do occur also reveal they are not universal. Such a mind/body connection is far less likely in animal experiments.

One animal study, interestingly, confirmed the high antiangiogenic power of a specially processed shark cartilage, the BeneFin brand. Researchers at the University of North Texas implanted 30 laboratory mice each with a lymphosarcoma tumor patch. Each mouse ingested 32 mg. daily of either bovine cartilage, a conventionally processed shark cartilage, or the BeneFin brand shark cartilage. While the segment of mice fed bovine cartilage showed no tumor necrosis, both shark cartilage counterparts did. The tumors were excised and cross-sectional photos were taken. These revealed that the greatest "Swiss cheese effect" occurred in the BeneFin-fed mice. This 1996 three-part experiment was small and had not been evaluated by the U.S. Food and Drug Administration. Yet its outcome was of such significance and its cost so low compared to the $30 billion already spent on cancer research, one must wonder why the experiment was not immediately replicated by other disinterested scientists.

Despite some shortcomings, John tends to place considerable credence in such studies. Because the medical establishment and related government bureaucracies have such monopolistic power, he feels the study is not likely to get a fair hearing. As to the argument that the results of this study has no significance for humans, it should be remembered that cross-sectional photos of tumors extracted from some who died in the Cuban study showed the same Swiss cheese appearance.

In a 1993 instructional video, “Shark Cartilage Therapy” (Information Services, Kerrville, Texas), a symposium of doctors from the New York Medical School was shown autopsy images of the malignant tumors excised from the five Cuban study subjects. The images showed not only the “Swiss cheese” necrosis caused by the shark cartilage but as well another unexpected outcome. While the tumors decayed from a lack of blood, fibrous connective tissue teeming with extra capillary networks simultaneously encapsulated them. A modulation of angiogenesis was noted! The host of the conference suggested this histological effect was “astonishing” and in light of all the evidence presented suggested the clinical effect of shark cartilage was “not explicable by chance.” A sidelight: one doctor had a prostate cancer patient with a PSA marker of 1700. Put on a hormone and shark cartilage simultaneously, the patient’s marker dropped to only 2.2 – and in just six weeks! The doctor had discussed this case with colleagues and none had ever heard of such a drop. Some conferees suggested a synergistic effect between the two therapies might have caused this 99 percent improvement. This was very encouraging because I too was on a hormonal and shark cartilage regimen.

But, alas, my CA-125 tumor marker of September 15, 1994, had actually risen 15 points. My oncologist and his intern didn’t despair because this rise to 113.0 was “still in the ball park” and no doubt an anomaly.

What a shock awaited me just down the road!

Lab Mice Tumor Medulla Comparison

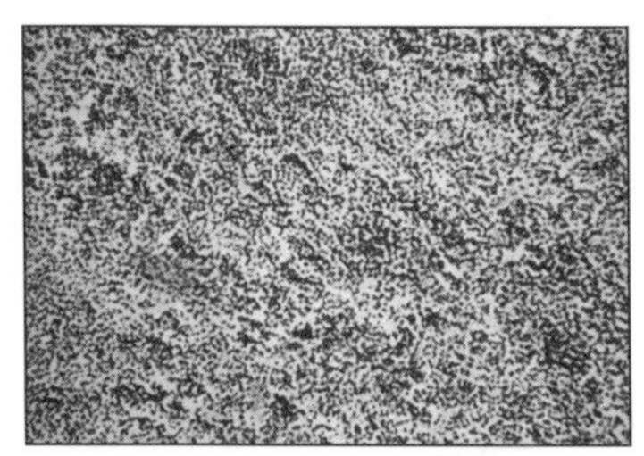

Bovine Cartilage (Control Specimen Similar). *No tumor necrosis observed.*

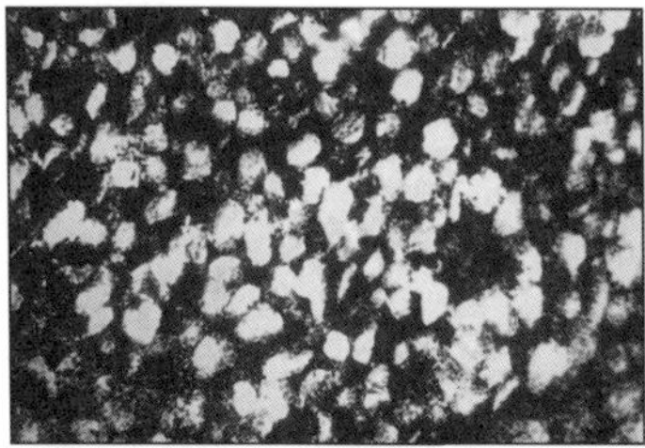

Organically Processed BeneFin Shark Cartilage *Extreme tumor necrosis (full "Swiss cheese effect").*

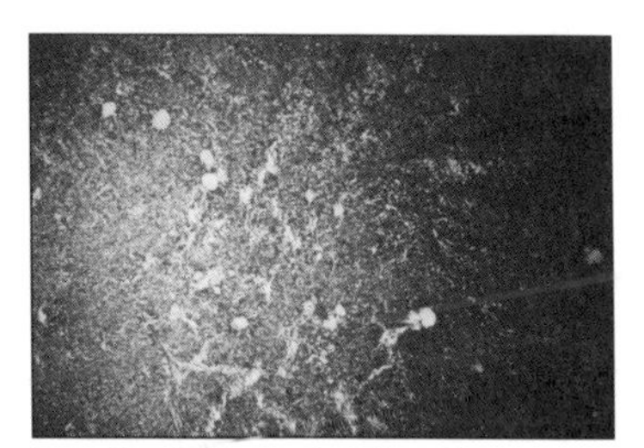

Leading Generic Shark Cartilage Product. *Considerable tumor necrosis (possible onset of "Swiss cheese effect") from antiangiogenesis.*

Microscopic slides courtesy of Lane Labs-USA, Inc., Allendale, NJ

The 1996 independent cancer study using 30 laboratory mice revealed that the daily ingestion of 32 mg. of shark cartilage did, indeed, result in tumor necrosis. The observed "Swiss cheese effect" was similar to the necrotic pattern of malignant tumors excised from human shark cartilage study participants. James R. Lott, Ph.D., Professor in Physiology at the University of North Texas, headed the animal experiment. Significantly, Dr. Lott's study had not been evaluated bythe U.S. Food and Drug Administration and apparently this low-cost experiment has not been repeated even once by others.

Later, I would come to wonder: Did my excised brain tumor exhibit this unique necrotic pattern?

chapter five

P-P-Panic!

Although the women behind the registration counter were busy shuffling papers, typing, and speaking to patients, the oncologist's office seemed cold and lifeless this brisk autumn day, November 2, 1994. And as we awaited my turn to see the doctor, I shivered briefly. I had now been on the shark cartilage some 14 or 15 weeks and had my blood drawn seven days earlier to determine my latest tumor marker which could by now show a positive response to the cartilage therapy. I tried to keep my thoughts reined in, but instead, they went wildly out of control. Finally, they locked onto what I could expect when sending John out with the weekly grocery list: every bag a surprise! And incredibly, I now found this memory so soothing that I was ready for anything... or so I thought.

When the nurse called us in I did feel composed. Soon, my doctor's new intern – very neat, very professional, very clinical – stepped in and cut short the usual pleasantries asking me numerous questions on how I felt, on whether any physical changes had been noticed, all the while shuffling through my voluminous records. I would be rotated from Tamoxifen to Megestrol, the usual with hormonal therapy. John asked, "How about the CA-125 marker?" Shuffling the papers again, the intern looked it up. "It was elevated," said he. "The lab is going to double check it." "But the number?" John persisted. "Exactly double the previous one, 226.0." At that moment, my oncologist stepped in and assured me that I wouldn't be alone and that there was hope. But already the roof had fallen in. I'll spare you an account of our ride home.

* * * *

The waving wind-blown grass, amber, crisp, strangely remote but beautiful, nodded, "You're home." As well, the first sounds of our driveway gravel beneath the tires offered soft somber notes. But the car doors slammed behind us and I could see that John was broken and all I could do was hug him and then fall into a long, fitful sleep.

The next morning I heard the words, "Were going to fight this." Miraculously, John was still trying to see through the cobwebs clouding my prospects. So intense was he that he had me sit down and started asking questions, even noting my responses on a pad! He asked me to describe the cancer pains and how they were different from the arthritis pain? What distinguishes the chemo pains from all the other pains? "Are you prepared for the fight of your life?" This last question resounded like a naughty thud! Was I? Of course! But the question, I realized, was always appropriate. It had become apparent to me that many people rather than face this kind of frightful anxiety readily capitulate to Death's final wish. I was not about to surrender and I cooperated with my benevolent questioner: Yes, the differences between the various pains were real and not in my pretty little head. John's chauvinism always seemed to emerge somehow but now it seemed so very reassuring and appropriate.

The dosages were next on John's agendum. A daily diary started July 12, 1994, the start of my shark cartilage regimen, now supplemented my somewhat more casual entries posted in a notebook and on calendars. Weekly dosage variations were thus revealed apparently caused by the gastrointestinal upsets influencing the amount of cartilage I actually measured especially for those portions taken orally. But still, precise calculations disclosed a daily average of 60.2 grams (excluding only the first four days of much lighter consumption meant to uncover possible side effects). But considering my depressed weight, it was close to the minimum generally recommended. Too, many of my retention enemas were being sustained well beyond the 30 minutes minimum. Happy faces neatly delineated the dates and times of these lofty accomplishments. Yes, these perspectives were from the pen of my husband whose appearance and temperament would suggest otherwise! And even more surprising, this husband of mine obtained the home phone number of Dr. I. William Lane.

It should be noted that my naturopathic physician had already been contacted and she suggested the 226 marker, although possibly an anomalous blip, might be the result of tumor mortification. A natural cancer treatment may cause a sharp marker rise because of a sudden outflow of the tumor's necrotic waste pulsing through the bloodstream toward evacuation. Even though a recent flu shot may have also had some influence, this explanation seemed reasonable to us.

Still, John was beside himself with worry and when he telephoned Lane's home and heard a powerful and impatient voice boom, "Bill Lane here, how may I help you?" he became muddled. But after an awkward start, John outlined my medical history and how my arthritis symptoms had disappeared. "I know the cartilage works!" Lane emphasized. "The important thing is to stay on track and make your wife well." He reminded John that cancer was a terrible scourge and it took time to treat. Then, it was John who was on the receiving end of questions.

In response to John's information, Lane said that I was using an effective brand of shark cartilage; that ingesting it orally was also effective; and that 15 weeks of cartilage therapy may be too early to determine its effectiveness. As to the 226 tumor marker spike? In his clinical trials, imaging was the primary assay and Lane offered no opinion except to say that the therapy appeared dosage sensitive and that late-stage cancer patients especially often increase their daily intake for a faster response time. He suggested we consider increasing my daily dosage level to 90 grams. (Also, he recommended a Tucson M.D. should we need additional medical consultation). I decided to increase my daily cartilage intake accordingly and now one dose was to be taken in the night. It was November 7, 1994, just five days following my last doctor visit, that I started this enhanced – and thus more difficult – regimen.

* * * *

Just days before, a deep voice, as though from the bowels of an open pit mine, rumbled into our lives. Telephoning us from his apartment just outside New York City, a retired security guard I'll call Barney asked for me as he was also on shark cartilage therapy. His burden was colorectal cancer also unresponsive to conventional modalities. Crude in both language and sentiment, he appeared to be an unlikely ally. But he and my husband formed quite a partnership born of mutual desperation. Also investigatory, Barney had telephoned the world's cancer and research centers for information including some in Australia and came to embrace shark cartilage therapy, but only tepidly. His was a dark and drizzly outlook. About our age and alone, his interest was in no halfway measure, but a full cure for the malignancy he little understood. He, however, appeared to be doing quite nicely, thank you, as his CEA tumor marker was down (from perhaps 700 or so) to only three!

It was actually a collaborative effort that had unearthed Dr. Lane's home telephone number and since Barney's condition seemed stabilized, my husband and he now plotted strategies for my care! For example, Barney reported that he had little trouble ingesting 110 grams of cartilage powder daily by taking it in four oral doses, each mixed with Diet Pepsi! Just the thought of such a combination was so repulsive that I decided to increase the number of my retention enemas from two daily to three and even though this change took more time, it made my enhanced regimen a bit easier. So I guess in this way, the collaboration was a help after all. But I was still taking three oral doses (not with Pepsi!), one of which was taken in the middle of the night for a more even distribution. John thought this "nocturnal caper" was a great idea for Barney, but he would have no part of it. He wanted to sleep.

Barney seemed buoyed by the exchanges he had with John and his tendency to shy from serious discussions with me strongly suggested a chauvinistic bent. Another reason, no doubt, the two men got on so well, at least at first.

To be sure, John has a suspicious nature but poor Barney appeared to be so paranoiac as to be largely dysfunctional. His questions as to why the medical community was so cool, if not hostile, toward natural therapies were thoughtful ones. And his law enforcement work no doubt helped him understand John's reasoning on the subject: that the big medical-pharmaceutical industry would rather not have the competition. In his work, he even saw that big money had a preponderant influence on government and other service agencies. My husband asked him if he had ever examined the JAMA, the Journal of the American Medical Association. He indeed had and also noticed its profusion of ads paid for by wealthy pharmaceutical companies. Barney had a world view similar to John's but his suspicion that the shark cartilage promotion was a scam nearly engulfed him. He could not come to a best guess and wholeheartedly run with it – as could John. This was the watershed that greatly distinguished these two.

Barney's story provides a number of tough lessons. On or about November 17, 1993, Barney was told by his doctors that all the chemotherapies he had endured did little to slow his cancer's progression. The malignancy had spread throughout his body but, fortunately, it was not that fast growing and thus he had perhaps a year to live. He started on the shark cartilage therapy about six months later, May or June of 1994. He telephoned us after about five months into his cartilage therapy. (He kept no records so his story is based on memory). About this time, his doctors started to take an increased interest in him apparently because he was still alive after a year and his tumor marker was so low. He had told them up front that he was going to start taking shark cartilage and while not particularly supportive they did not try to dissuade him.

His doctors did not credit the shark cartilage for his improved condition, only suggesting a delayed reaction to the chemotherapy was a possibility. Thoroughly bewildered, Barney became more and more uncertain and soon his tumor markers inched up a little and he underwent – again, from the description he gave us – an onocostint scan. It revealed that the larger tumors had now become "little spots." Instead of being heartened over this good news, he took it as a sign of failure because the tumors were still there.

At this point, he told John that he was giving up and not returning to his doctors anymore. After a long talk with my husband, Barney did return to receive some of the same chemotherapy that had previously failed and his tumor markers marched smartly downward! John was ecstatic about this news but Barney still complained that the cartilage had not been a complete cure.

Partly from noting Barney's attitude and its apparent physical ramifications, my husband now came to fully understand that there is indeed a crucial mind/body connection and it can mean the difference between life and death and it had an effect on <u>his</u> outlook. John started encouraging me to watch some of instructional videos again that I had found so reassuring and started talking about my joining a support group. John broached the subject of joining a support group with Barney, but Barney responded, "I don't wanna."

* * * *

Barney's bulldog tenacity did provide considerable information and inspired John to call the 800 number of the National Cancer Institute to see what information might be had concerning the CA-125 tumor marker. The warm voice answering the phone did not in the least sound like that of a bureaucrat. The woman listened attentively as John briefly outlined my case and the troubling tumor marker of 226. This call was made one day following a blood draw for the next marker. It was November 30, 1994, and

John was very worried that more bad news would be forthcoming. He immediately opened up and expressed just how worried he was even though all other signs indicated the shark cartilage was working.

To his surprise, she seemed to suggest that these other indicators had weight and that the tumor marker was not perfect. It could be thrown off by a number of conditions and that one should look for a pattern over a number of months, she instructed. John had gotten the impression she was a nurse and perhaps new to the job as she spent an hour on the phone and seemed interested in learning about this cartilage I was taking. She offered to mail a full listing of formal clinical trials now in the offing just in case the cartilage failed. The bulging package came a few days later.

Scores of notices were included, written in a language meant for doctors. A medical dictionary and two or three days of concentration brought disappointment. Virtually all were variations of old conventional therapies obviously put there in hopes of expanding their ranges and thus company profits. Regardless, with all their restrictive protocols, even the chance of finding one in time was not all that likely. We had made up our minds that my best hope lay in the alternative arena and even began allowing our many conventional journal subscriptions to expire. We felt that any conventional breakthroughs of significance would be included in the alternative writings and, accordingly, our subscription habits changed.

It was I who had always accepted manipulation therapies as well as social and psychological support mechanisms. Even though John tended to view these as "fluff," he had agreed to my having shiatsu treatments given by a licensed local practitioner who came to the home. This finger pressure therapy had started back several months before Barney's dismal outlook and its obvious medical consequences had influenced John's thinking on such matters. Thus, at first, he tended to eye this "acupressure" approach with reserve as its ethereality did not mesh with his more earthy instincts.

The leg distress and gastrointestinal upsets were but two components of my discomfort. At times, another outgrowth of past chemotherapy locked my back in a dull and sometimes excruciating pain. Once, John offered to massage the spinal area and it brought considerable relief. The shiatsu therapy, I thought, was a logical and precise progression from John's more ponderous efforts. And it seemed to help.

Because the back pain centered in the area just behind the stomach, both my naturopathic physician and the shiatsu practitioner hypothesized a nerve connection from the stomach. Whatever the theory, the treatments decreased the pain and were relaxing. Most often, though, the pain returned within a few hours but did provide time for a more restful nap. But following one treatment, I was without pain for 13 days!

After this hiatus, the pain did return but was less severe. One technique I was taught involved my making a closed fist and pressing it in a rolling motion over and around the gastrointestinal area to stimulate the normal motions of the stomach and intestinal tract. This technique was an especial aide as it helped move the food along by increasing the peristaltic action which is modulated by the autonomic nervous system. Significantly, the abdominal area felt less pliable than normal and both my N.D. and the practitioner sensed the possibility of future problems. The practitioner taught John some pressure points to use which also helped but after about 10 months the pain subsided enough that the therapy was no longer needed. With the digestive enzymes, herbs, and other nutritional supplements prescribed by the N.D., I was doing well enough – at least, at that time.

But it was Pearl Harbor Day, December 7, 1994, that I knew would be a day portending either massive wreckage or my survival. My blood draw for the next CA-125 tumor marker had been taken eight days before this date – this date which was looming just ahead and accelerating my anxiety. It was, of course, my next office visit to see my oncologist.

In an attempt to offset my apprehension, I kept busy, however fitfully, and found myself putting an audio tape into our cassette player. Its title: "Dr. I. William Lane's WOR Radio Interveiw With Joan Hamburg" (Information Services, Kerrville, Texas). The call-in program not only featured an interview with Dr. Lane, but opened with the co-editor of "60 Minutes," Mike Wallace, on the telephone. Wallace remarked on how suspicious he was in the beginning but became less so as the Cuban clinical trial progressed. He came to realize that "No doubt, there is some validity to his (Lane's) thesis." He also noted that experts enlisted to help in the investigation drew similar conclusions. His observation that early on the Cuban patients experienced a reduction in pain and a heightened sense of well-being was also encouraging as those same benefits had managed to pierce through my underlying anxiety and the aftereffects of the chemotherapy.

We had listened to this audio tape some months earlier and we were amazed how even this short lapse of time had changed our overall perception of it. Now, the content of the program and the fact that Mike Wallace even bothered to call in seemed all the more astonishing. We again heard Dr. Lane suggest that if it hadn't been for his promotional efforts, the preliminary studies on cartilage, though published, probably would have been ignored for many decades. John nodded in full agreement.

That same day, December 6, I rummaged through some copies of my medical records and started reading an account of the surgery and initial diagnosis and it served as a stark reminder of my life's fragility.

The report began:

PREOPERATIVE DIAGNOSIS: Pelvic *mass.*

POSTOPERATIVE DIAGNOSIS: Cancer of the ovary and cancer of the endometrium. Stage pending final pathology.

OPERATION PERFORMED: 1. By Dr. Dxxxx: Total abdominal hysterectomy, bilateral salpingo-oophorectomy.

2. By Dr. Hxxxx: Pelvic and para-aortic node biopsies. Omentectomy, biopsy of paritoneal surface of mesoappendix, biopsy of right hemidiaphragm, biopsy of right paracolic gutter, resection of retroperitoneal tumor in the pelvic cul-de-sac.

Tomorrow I should know whether all the efforts by my doctors and my husband will be brought to naught by this sneaky onset of Stage III malignancies.

chapter six

What?

Actually, death was not on my mind when I awoke and made ready for the 10:15 AM doctor appointment. John, though, was somber. This December 7th seemed quite like any other day as the media hadn't much noted the Japanese sneak attack on Pearl Harbor as the intervening years in 1994 carried an off number. It's 50th anniversary in '91 by contrast had had pre-eminent media regard. But still, my own prospects might be in for another shock on this date which forevermore would live "in infamy." What will come will come thought I so that my mind should dwell elsewhere. But as we left the elevator on the second floor of the building whose form had been etched by so many visits, the tapping of my pumps echoed. I imagined a metallic tone the likes of which might have echoed down the corridors of those vessels now twisted beneath the shallow harbor water. The death of so many innocent young men pressed against me and I slowed down. And into the office we stepped. The now familiar women behind the registration counter were still quiet in shuffling papers, typing, speaking to patients. And again muted, we awaited my turn. John was still so very somber.

The WOR radio program I had again listened to just 20 hours before filtered into my thoughts. One middle aged woman named Frankie had been discussed. Her ovarian tumor initially weighed over 30 pounds and in a way this Cuban study participant was fortunate that by feel alone the tumor shrinkage was evident. Here I sat with comparatively small tumors and had to deal with the anxiety of not knowing with certainty that the cartilage was performing as hoped. And I had been on full dosages of the powder for nearly 20 weeks and we well knew that within such time if solid evidence doesn't surface, this might indicate the prospect of little or no benefit. This thought lingered as we were called into the examination room. Strangely, I again felt completely composed but I could see that John was doing less well.

It was worse being in such a small room and John's ruddy and tan features now turned decidedly ashen. Some distant voices were heard mingled with abrupt laughs. A single set of rather light footsteps suddenly became apparent and a young wiry intern burst into the room with my folder held just above the shoulder line as if too heavy to carry otherwise. He quickly introduced himself and then asked a number of now familiar questions all the while keeping his eyes fixed on us. Not once did he refer to the folder and he had just a hint of smile that somehow suggested a compressed spring ready to be released.

But the medical probes continued until John, himself a bit flustered by all the kinetic energy filling the room, asked about the blood test result. "Forty-five point two" said he, enunciating each syllable with eyes twinkling with just a hint of disbelief perhaps combined with expectation. "What?" "Forty-five point two." John and I turned to each other and in unison exclaimed, "It's the shark cartilage!" With a quick bounce the intern smiled and excused himself racing out and leaving the door partly open.

Within seconds, the booming voice of my oncologist filled the little room. "So, it's the shark cartilage!" he said, then turning to the intern who was now peering into my voluminous folder. "It is definitely ovarian cancer," the intern mumbled as though asking for confirmation. "Yes," my oncologist said. Then abruptly becoming the instructor, he faced the intern and noted the international animal and human trials along with the nearby test tube experiments at the University of Arizona Health Science Center, that suggest shark cartilage may possess antiangeogenic tumor fighting power. My oncologist then turned to us saying that this drop from 226 in less than five weeks was unexpected and impressive and that I should continue taking the cartilage. "Just continue whatever you're doing, " he counseled. "We don't want to shoot this gift horse in the mouth."

As we paid our bill and turned to leave, the jovial intern held up the book, *Sharks Don't Get Cancer* and said that another patient had brought it in. As we left, we had the feeling some sort of betting may have been going on. Even the women behind the counter were paying attention and generally evincing good humor. And John looked relieved.

* * * *

One must understand that John is one of those persons who tends to examine a conclusion he deems critical until all contraindications, however meager, are explored if not toppled. I had concluded that the latest marker of 45.2 was not only of itself a weighty indicator but coupled with my doctor's reaction to it a decisive one. After all, this was about an 80 percent drop! And just within five weeks. Even Barney exclaimed, "Y-e-a-h, g-r-e-a-t!!" Such jubilation surprised us owing to his previously persistent melancholy. But this husband of mine, while relieved, still questioned the accuracy of the CA-125 tumor marker. Thus a-probing he went.

We had been buying the cartilage from a New York City physician's supply outlet that housed a pharmacy. John had had a number of telephone conversations with the chief pharmacist there and decided to call him about my latest experience. He did not seem surprised by my roller coaster ride as he felt that the marker was only a rough indicator, at least for some people. He explained that those undergoing cartilage therapy are often in the final stages of their cancer and that x-rays or other imaging techniques are thus most often used. It was his impression, however, that tumor markers behaved differently with natural therapies. Also, the marker is a measure of past events and, consequently, its revelations always run late, he concluded.

This last bit of information was unfamiliar and John started cogitating: If a sudden rise in the tumor marker does indicate a positive breakdown of tumors and this was reflected belatedly, then there was a closer correspondence between the marker and my earlier subjective improvements, especially the disappearance of the painful abdominal pressure after just seven weeks on the cartilage therapy.

Of course John knew that this was speculative and so he called the NCI 800 number again and told the woman who answered about my case and that he was trying to determine the validity and reliability of the CA-125 tumor marker. He told her of his considerable reading on the marker but could not find any formal large-scale studies. And then a barrage of questions followed: What evidence is there that a set of discrete marker numbers have real world correlates, say the stages of the corresponding malignancies determined by other means? Does the marker work well with most patients? How might one determine if it is working in my wife's case? Is empiricism the only avenue used to justify its use?

It was obvious that the receiving end was bewildered. The poor women agreed that the marker, although used extensively, was known to register inaccuracies but that she herself knew little about it and would consult a colleague who might. If she uncovered any more information that might be useful, she would call back. John murmured something about medicine involving a lot of guesswork and that he doubted that a response would be forthcoming. He was right.

John decided that we had to work with what was out there and again sat down with me to analyze, step by step, the vital events of my case. Finally, he concluded the cartilage was most likely working. Now, I could have told him that and with a lot less trouble!

* * * *

Probability and levels of confidence play central roles in

nailing down a conclusion or course of action. This is my husband pure and simple. Intuition and gut feelings are part of the mix but are almost always suspect. A just-the-facts mentality dominates. Something like an elephant standing in the middle of the living room, you know it's there.

This is not to say he is a beast... not quite. He has a non-analytical side as well but cooler embers tend to obscure its warmth. In gathering material for this writing, I came upon the *Bride's Reference Book* published by Bride's House Incorporated in 1953. "From the day you say 'I do,' your home and your husband come first," is the lead sentence of one of its chapters. I had some rather hearty laughs at this and similar sentiments tucked away for so long in its yellowed pages. John, though, responded differently. "Remember when you told your second graders that at the time you had been married 35 years and one little boy asked, 'To the same man?'" He then fondly reflected on the little girl next door who would come over and visit. This was soon after we were married and the little girl and I would talk and sort of play – that is, until he got home and I had to stop to fix dinner. "Divorce him, but keep Prince" was her suggested remedy. Prince was our dog. Outside of her humorous priorities, we remembered this event so well because divorce was less common then and the subject seldom came up. How times have changed.

Later, I came upon John gently binding the book's frayed cover with clear tape. Perhaps I should have responded to it differently as I realized that the permanence of our marriage may have been the critical difference offering me hope and the chance to live with John just the way he is. Having strong anchors to the past is sometimes admirable. (In keeping with this sentiment it should be mentioned that we are still in contact with the girl and her parents who have been married 58 years! Their daughter is married and has two lovely girls.)

So how did this warm-hearted husband of mine use cold logic to estimate the efficacy of the cartilage I was now taking? Here's how: he and Barney were at it again and somehow secured the office telephone number of the first NCI-trained cancer expert enlisted by the producers of "60 Minutes." The information thus obtained was added to that information already garnered and this better enabled John to evaluate each therapeutic event in terms of probability. His estimates follow: the probability that it was the action of the cartilage that wiped out my arthritis symptoms: 90 percent; the chance that the cartilage eliminated the painful abdominal pressure: 80 percent; the probability that the cartilage was responsible for an increased feeling of well being: 40 percent; the chance that the shark cartilage was mainly responsible for the big drop in the CA-125 tumor marker: 80 percent. One could reasonably conclude that there was a very high probability that the total therapeutic result was not the result of chance. Of course, John knows that such estimates must always be viewed with some caution but he felt his estimates were actually conservative. He had also determined that the hormonal treatment was essentially a holding action but may have made its contribution synergistically.

John tried to explain all this to Barney but he remained in a funk, his recent jubilant expressions not withstanding.

* * * *

Despite having suffered a mild cold the first part of December, I was feeling somewhat better and even decided on a Christmas trip to meet with relatives near Prescott, Arizona some 250 miles north of us. John felt that my therapeutic regimen including the retention enemas should be maintained while on the trip. At this time we were not sure that the retention enemas were an essential element of my therapy but we were disinclined to take chances. Yet, as one might imagine, I was not enthralled about tying up one of the two bathrooms for at least 30 minutes three times a day, especially with so many of us in the home.

Grandma Florence, the then 78-year-old mother of my former

sister-in-law, Jackie, had moved from the Chicago area to Prescott just the previous summer. She had settled in a manufactured home park nestled among an old stand of magnificent pine in a beautiful rock-studded mountainous region just outside the city. Besides Grandma, John and I, Jackie and her two daughters, Susan and Kerria, would be there. Of course, the details of my therapy were explained to one and all, and it was obvious that it didn't matter. "I'm sure John will keep you on schedule," Jackie laughed.

And on schedule I was. With John's help, elaborate plans were made even for the seven-hour drive there. The ill effects of the past chemotherapy, though diminished slightly, were still unrelievedly present and we had to stop frequently especially for vigorous walks not only to relieve the intermittent pain of my left leg but to help prevent its forming another clot. Also, the gastrointestinal upsets were mitigated by John's roadside back massages. We made it without incident and even stopped at a delightfully rustic restaurant along the way. And I was actually able to eat something! Not a whole meal by any means, but a greater amount than what had become usual. True to form, I was so happy to have actually made it to Grandma's home and so engrossed in family discourse that some of those times set aside for taking the cartilage would have glided by had it not been for John. Often, I could divine an appointed hour just by his posture. I answered each and every call, save one. Quite good, thought I, since I was still taking 90 plus grams per day in six dosages. One event that somewhat dampened the six-day holiday, however, was the cold rainy weather. The other was concern for our little dog who, while under the care of a very attentive neighbor, was still suffering from separation anxiety. When we arrived home our worst fears were confirmed as Coco had spent her days quietly crying and testing the cool northern air searching for us.

* * * *

Coco had some of our old bedding and the melodious sounds

of a familiar radio station for comfort, but John decided that for this dog it wasn't enough and he had an idea that he said would cleverly assuage the problem and at the same time foster a towering level of community spirit. I listened to his plan with some skepticism. Needless to say, I have seen some of his "clever" projects come crashing down around him. I'm speaking both literally and figuratively. Thus, when he comes up with an idea that seems to strain the limits of sanity, I smile and wonder.

Just days before our next trip, he telephoned our neighbors and described in considerable detail the travails our dog goes through when denied extensive humanoid contact. Many of the neighbors jog, walk, horseback ride and otherwise enjoy the beautiful countryside and agreeable climate. He suggested that while they were out they might enjoy communing with this lovable dog of ours and were encouraged to come by for a canine visit. And it worked! People came from far and near and were sometimes bumping into one another. One grandmother actually thanked us for keeping her in mind as her granddaughter just loved coming over. Others attached Coco's leash and took her along on their walks. In this case, John latched onto something. A lonely dog did provide the catalyst for a kind of lofty community involvement and, interestingly, Coco's separation anxiety had all but disappeared.

Human character can have its dark side but the magnanimity shown by so many for such a small creature reminds one of its great potential for beauty and warmth. I had met so many fine spirits who helped inspire my continued survival. Neighbors, nurses, doctors, pharmacists, business people and, yes, even strangers whom I had met but fleetingly have made it obvious that not all on this planet are insensitive. To be sure, I did encounter some blots. But it is the perfidious type which may at times fully blight the landscape. It didn't take long to realize that the terminally ill are often discouraged by a sly prejudice. And the "upstanding" persons so involved may come as a revelation to those uninitiated in the wayward behavior of a cartel.

As has already been mentioned, there is some tension between John and me because we sometimes perceive things differently. Much of this difference comes from the fact that women of my generation often were not exposed to the more unseemly aspects of life. In other words, by design and deed, like most women, I was protected. Now John immediately discerned that something was seriously amiss in the health care field and almost imediately sensed that a cartel prevailed and distorted health care to a point that the patient in many ways stood to be the loser.

John and I were not reared in a sterling metropolis filled with innocence and good will. While the Chicago metropolitan region is noted for its windy political figures and great cultural and economic resources, it is perhaps less well known for its "shadow governments" made up of people of questionable character. A kind of monopoly imposed on business. These mob types were hardly personages in the refined sense, but they did the things one would expect of a cartel. But at that time a woman was not likely to have the kind of experiences that would make this apparent to her. Let me cite one example.

John's father owned businesses in Chicago and had considerable contact with this element and was privy to their methods. Interestingly, they openly battled one another but used more subtle techniques in keeping the ordinary working people – almost all men – in line. These included physical threats but only occasionally. Once, John's father hired an independent trucker to haul away the business-generated trash. Soon, city inspectors were all over him and he realized that to keep his business licenses he would have to pay the extra cost of an "approved" hauler. The free-lance hauler was also threatened and ultimately gave up this sideline.

The main surprise in this was that for weeks following this forced capitulation, John's father received phone calls and visits from aldermen and others of such rank warmly congratulating him on his upstanding citizenship! To be sure, I had heard this account many years ago but tended to recoil from it, as I do now. On the other hand, my husband having also been in the cold business world for a time finds it easy to incorporate this and other such information in his frame of reference.

* * * *

Our distant memories help provide us with the foundation for this present effort in still other ways. We well remember the days of the Great Depression. We remember when a doctor was a neighbor who made house calls and might be found staying the night to attend a sick child. We also remember that most people depended on health tips handed down over the generations and we can speak from experience in suggesting that these remedies seemed to have helped. We remember, too, the low-tech doctor's bag housing a thermometer, tongue depressors and a flashlight to probe the throat. And now I fondly remember tilting my head back, mouth opened wide, and resonating what so many of my generation had uttered, "a-a-a-a-w."

No smiling, please. This essentially was all that was available and continuing hardship was usually the norm as you can see from brief examples from our own early medical history. John weighed 10 pounds 12 ounces at birth and thus became a black-and-blue "instrument baby." This trauma was followed by potentially fatal childhood diseases including whooping cough and rheumatic fever which left him for a time with a damaged heart. I was born prematurely and weighed under five pounds but my mother and I were released from the hospital since there was nothing to do but wait and hope. Convulsions soon followed and I was treated by a savvy older woman who quickly dipped me in warm water and brought the spasms under control just in time to regain my breath. This prompt action was credited by the doctor with saving my life. This kind neighbor was not disparaged by the doctor nor arrested for practicing medicine. Nor did she have to worry about being sued as the number of lawyers back then was low and most of those were true neighbors. Apparently, I was allergic to normal breast feeding and when I was put on goats' milk the convulsions vanished. Chicken pox, measles, and the other normal childhood diseases came and went but I managed to live on to face the mother of all diseases, cancer, and not only did I write home about it but as well decided to compose this chronicle of love and hope.

chapter seven

Head Tremors and The Unforeseen

The year of 1995 spanned an improbable series of events any one of which could have caused my death. As pivotal as this year was, its beginning saw but minor turbulences that obscured the major storms lurking in the mist ahead. It was the proverbial lull.

On our way home from Prescott we stopped for my blood draw which registered a slightly elevated CA-125 tumor marker. It had risen almost six points to 50.9, a seemingly minor rise, but still my oncologist in the next office visit January 4, 1995, seemed to be oblivious to the high excitement of my previous appointment, responding with a lilting "h-m-m h-m-m" and a shuffling of my records as I tried to talk about the cartilage. Then, he suggested continuing the hormonal treatment, 160 mg. of Megace daily, and to start a per diem intake of some aspirin to help forestall further blood clotting in my troublesome left leg. But as he moved to leave John said, "Her arthritis symptoms have disappeared." And John had his full attention. My oncologist evidently knew of this beneficial effect of shark cartilage therapy, yet now appeared edgy discussing it.

Five days later, I switched to the second generation of clinical grade shark cartilage which is processed in Australia using a chemical free enzymatic method. Thus, this new BeneFin brand shark cartilage had fewer of its bioactive macro proteins damaged or destroyed. Besides having a high 44 percent protein content, it was somewhat cleaner both in smell and taste which, unfortunately, made little difference. Even after all these months taking it, I had not gotten used to the powder's odd, fishy taste. And although somewhat improved in this regard, the new brand carried this taste tradition forward quite admirably. It would be many more months before an improved orange flavored variety would be introduced. But I still make a bit of a face in taking this new flavor. Not so fondly, I still hear echoes of my dear husband saying, "Just take it and keep quiet."

The selection of my new primary care internist months earlier proved auspicious as from the start he teamed well with my oncologist and generally inspired our confidence. On my fourth visit, I made efforts to bring him up to date on my cartilage therapy but his questions and medical probes were ascendant and my words lost out in the exchange. So after a time, John caught a quiet moment and said, "Her arthritis has disappeared." The doctor opened his eyes wide and crossed his fingers. "It's often a beneficial side effect of the cartilage," John said as he started to repeat what I had been trying to report. The doctor appeared ruffled, but John plowed forward. Fortunately, he kept the account brief and the internist turned reflective and suggested that taming rheumatoid arthritis was not easy. He then asked John to provide him with copies of whatever materials were pertinent as he was interested in learning more. Thus, my initial impression was reinforced. Intuitively, I knew I had made a wise choice in selecting this particular HMO doctor. Strangely, though, his interest in the cartilage centered more on the control of arthritis than cancer! But for me the cancer reined.

* * * *

Each bodily change, each recurrence of a symptom, each respiratory infection, each "whatever" grabbed my attention because of its possible connection to the malignancy. True, much of what I endured was by now familiar, especially the gastrointestinal upsets. Still, there were surprises even with these repeaters. A difference in the duration, the severity, or even the time of an occurrence signaled a possible connection to the cancer. Some of the problems seemed alien. Once my right thumb developed an unusual hour-long pain only for it to vanish. Later, my left knee developed a brief pain that moved to the other knee and just as quickly disappeared. And the nature of these errant pains was unlike that of my old arthritic torments.

The gastrointestinal distress which emerged so regularly became the target of a test I devised to see if a change in diet would lessen the pain. The shark cartilage, I had already determined, did worsen the upsets but only slightly and, of course, eliminating the cartilage from the oral portion of my regimen was not a likely option. I could not see myself being solely dependent on retention enemas because of the additional time required. Consequently, even though I had been told that these stomach upsets were almost certainly the result of the very toxic chemotherapy I had had, I felt that by briefly eliminating certain foods or supplements one at a time, an aggravator might be uncovered. But none was revealed except for the garlic capsules which I had already suspected and thus was going to discontinue taking anyway. Fortunately, I found that a small amount of this healthful food cooked with a meal was well tolerated. In the end, however, the elimination of the garlic capsules helped little.

A little later, the addition of acidophilus capsules to my diet did help significantly by taking the edge off of the stomach upsets and reducing the vomiting and retching. Each capsule contains millions of specially cultivated live bacteria that sometimes help restore the favorable balance of the intestinal flora. It was the New York pharmacist mentioned earlier who recommended it.

Although periodic cold infections had sometimes spanned my other more frequent ailments, on the whole my condition seemed to be improving. Therefore, when I was to see my oncologist February 15, 1995, my biggest worry revolved around the next tumor marker.

* * * *

John and I arrived early for the 11 AM appointment and it was still apparent that the incessant drip of uncertainty was wearing on both of us. It was I, however, who was the most unsettled on this rather frigid morning. I didn't know what to expect. John was also worried but typically he manages a somewhat more even keel. Still, worry bathed his countenance as well.

When beckoned to have my weight taken and for both of us to proceed to an examining room, all the familiar sounds seemed just a bit hollow. I could feel urgent pulses in my left arm as the nurse took my blood pressure, yet the pressure was in the normal range. My oncologist's voice seemed softer than usual as he happily entered the room. His countenance aglow, he turned to report a tumor marker of 76.2, elevated some 25 points, but still good news. "Nothing to worry about at this stage," he said.

I wondered. But the doctor's positive demeanor quickly dispelled much of my doubt. John also brightened. After asking a series of questions on how I was feeling (to which I had mostly positive answers), my oncologist immediately turned to John. During an earlier visit, the doctor had mentioned knowing one of the nearby shark cartilage researchers and it was obvious he held this researcher in high esteem. Now, he again mentioned this researcher's work as if to set the stage for all the questions he was about to ask John. And the questions tumbled out in quick succession.

He wanted to know what made John think there might be an effective experimental treatment "out there" to begin with. There were a few questions about the methods John used in gathering information, but most of the doctor's inquiries centered on what difficulties might have been encountered in buying the cartilage itself. After John explained that he had a rather easy time finding a reliable source, a physician's supply outlet in New York City, the doctor's response was revealing. " So you didn't have to prowl some dark alley to find it," he said while smiling even more broadly than before. As the session came to a close, it was obvious to both of us that my oncologist knew more about cartilage therapy than we were giving him credit for and that he somehow discerned that despite the somewhat elevated tumor marker, the cartilage was working. This last assessment was strengthened four weeks later when the tumor marker dropped to 68.1, some eight points lower. Some relief was in the air.

* * * *

Relief or not, there are times I can't explain my behavior. For example, I am usually prompt in making a necessary doctor's appointment, unlike John who must often be pushed and prodded. But for whatever reason I kept putting off making an appointment to see my primary care physician as had been earlier requested. And, now, it was John who was doing the pushing and prodding and becoming angrier by the day as I procrastinated. Finally, he was going to make the call himself. At that point I relented and agreed to pick up the phone. John pointed out that unless I had a specific medical complaint the wait might be two or three months and thus suggested mentioning a head tremor that I had recently developed. We both knew that such a tremor is often the result of chemotherapy but, nonetheless, I mentioned the complaint and received an earlier appointment day, March 8, 1995. And how providential this casual afterthought became!

When my doctor came into the examining room he aimed for my head, literally. He pressed on it, tried to hold it still, and felt all around the back of it. His examination was intense. Then he had me do a series of exercises to test my coordination and balance. Then we heard what we expected to hear, that the cause was probably the side effect of the carboplatin, which often causes permanent nerve damage. Then the unexpected was said, "Just to be sure, we better schedule an MRI scan." At the time we thought my internist was just being thorough which trait appeared to be basic to his nature. We both thought that he might have trouble convincing the HMO of the scan's necessity. And our premonition was correct.

It didn't take but several days to learn that my HMO had decided against the MRI scan. My primary care doctor said that he was going to resubmit the request with some additional corroboration. He felt that the scan was necessary given my medical history and the fact that the tremors and certain other symptoms do suggest the possibility of causes outside of the chemotherapy. "There is a 95 percent chance that it will go through," he said.

"In the event it doesn't, we'll have the scan done outside of the HMO," John said. For whatever reason my doctor seemed somewhat insulted by this and emphasized that he would vigorously challenge the HMO's decision. "It is medically necessary," he emphasized.

The fact that this unexpected concern over my head tremors may have resulted from my procrastination in making the office appointment in the first place was not lost on us. Perhaps the doctor would have zeroed in on the tremors anyway, but still, the appointment time would have been delayed by at least a month if I hadn't mentioned it when phoning for the appointment. In a matter of days we were informed that the MRI scan was approved and scheduled for the Monday afternoon of March 20, 1995. Even though there was some tension in the air stemming from the rejection and then the sudden and unexplained rush to have the MRI performed, John and I felt no apprehension. In fact, I was amused by the whole process.

The technician first informed me that the scan was very noisy and would last 20 minutes and then asked if I had a favorite music station that I would like to hear to help pass the time. I chose a public classical music station but the beautiful music piped through earplugs was eerily distorted by the frenzied mechanical sounds that bombarded the tight chamber I was in. Talk about incongruity! It was a relief to have the cacophony end!

Quite happily I anticipated getting dressed and doing some late shopping when I was somberly met by both the radiologist and the technician as I emerged from the chamber. They minced no words in telling me that the scan showed a four-centimeter tumor putting critical pressure on my cerebellum or brain stem. In fact, they had already called my primary care physician and they told me to see him as soon as possible. My world now was upside down and even getting dressed took on a surrealistic slowness and by the time I met John in the waiting room all hope of beating this terrible cancer had drained from my body.

* * * *

The news had hit John harder than it would have had he not been under the misconception that shark cartilage tended to be less effective in treating brain tumors. He had been in contact with the East Coast office of one of the "60 Minutes" medical consultants and had learned that shark cartilage therapy seemed to be less effective with some types tumors. But in checking his notes John realized that brain tumors did not fall in this category. This realization bolstered his spirits considerably.

It goes without saying, nevertheless, that John was very nervous and agitated and it showed when we met with my primary care physician at 9:00 AM two days later.

My doctor had squeezed us between his regular appointments this Wednesday morning and thus he rushed into the examination room somewhat out of breath. "I'm sorry to have to tell you that the outlook appears bleak," were his first hurriedly spoken words. But when he saw John's reaction the doctor slowed down and explained that the tumor was probably metastatic and even if removed some of the malignancy would remain and likely grow and spread. "Most likely, we would only be buying some time," he concluded.

It was obvious by John's tight, steely reaction that he wasn't accepting any of this and the doctor took a deep breath and held out the possibility that my tumor wasn't related to the ovarian cancer and could possibly be benign. "But that is only a long shot," he cautioned.

"I think the shark cartilage has been working," John said. My internist looked at him with a profoundly perplexed expression, as did I, frankly. The doctor then discussed percentages which showed my prognosis appeared very bleak, indeed.

Still, John revealed that he had some other experimental treatment programs lined up for me should this worst case scenario prove true. My internist shook his head ever so slightly and suggested that such an approach while understandable will likely lead to a waste of both time and money. But it was obvious that John was not swayed.

* * * *

Again, one must remember that although I had been feeling slightly better, the continuing effects of my past chemotherapy sapped my energy and thus I could not vigorously participate in any of these discussions. Therefore, I tended to sit quietly with my hands folded. On top of it, John's tenacity tends to be overpowering. This was especially evident when we met with the neurosurgeon the next morning.

The brain surgeon came highly recommended as being one of the very best in the City of Tucson and when we met him we could understand why as he exuded the kind of supreme confidence that can only come from one having consumate skill and knowing it. Middle aged, soft-spoken and calm, he seemed to us to represent the quintessential surgeon. But it didn't take long for the poor surgeon to become unraveled.

John didn't say much during the surgeon's rather lengthy explanations of the MRI images and how they revealed imminent danger. "The pressure against the brain stem could result in death at any time and we must prepare for surgery without delay," he said. Then he explained that the tumor's removal would only buy some time as it was "virtually certain" to be metastatic and, consequently, terminal. It was at this point that John tried to explain the various aspects of my shark cartilage therapy and how he thought it was working. "If I don't miss my guess, the antiangiogenic effects of the cartilage will be apparent when you cut into the tumor," John said to the now quite baffled surgeon. Lost for words, the surgeon stared blankly at the two of us for some little time before turning and asking me to enumerate all of the things I was taking, which I did. As I progressed, trying to remember everything, it was apparent that the surgeon's blood pressure was rising. Finally, he exclaimed, "Health food stuff! Get off of everything! Your system must be clear of all of these things before surgery." John explained that I had already stopped taking the cartilage several days ago so that its antiangiogenic powers wouldn't interfere with surgery or subsequent healing. We were told to return to his office the next day, as the surgeon was going to order some extra tests and a second MRI scan needed to guide surgical preparations and then he turned to John and again reminded him of the seriousness of my condition. It was obvious to me that John remained hard of hearing not only literally (he wears a hearing aid) but figuratively as well.

* * * *

It should be noted that during this very stressful period much of our time was spent not only seeing my doctors but going to the Tucson labs for various blood tests and other procedures in preparation for my brain surgery and we had little time to absorb the events let alone discuss them. Much of the time we were on autopilot.

Yet I was alert enough to sense that something could go wrong because of the time constraints. In fact, I told the technician taking my blood draws that it was important to double check everything as I was due for critical brain surgery in the matter of a day or so. Unbelievably, one of the blood tests was omitted and I had to return to the lab early the following day for another blood draw less than 24 hours before my scheduled surgery!

Immediately following the blood draw I had to go in to have my head prepared. Little "Life Savors" were cemented to my head to provide radiological reference points to help guide the surgeon through this very delicate surgery. The technician provided me with a mirror and the little rings made me look like a creature from outer space. She went on to explain how I would be placed on the operating table stomach down with my head tightly clamped in a rigid metal ring to prevent any chance of it moving during the procedure. And when John and I went in to see the surgeon and learned that I was to be at the hospital at 5:30 AM sharp the next day, Saturday, March 25, I can't say I was up to speed. But I had made up my mind that I would stay alert and express whatever concerns I might have.

The surgeon reminded me of the imminent danger caused by the pressure against the brain stem and thus of the reason for the early morning schedule. Then displaying a number of forms, he very softly enumerated some of the possible outcomes of the surgery: full or partial paralysis; a comatose state; or even death. He outlined these possibilities on the various forms and had me sign them. While warm and sympathetic, it was obvious that he wanted no misunderstandings – that even though I might survive a very delicate and dangerous procedure, my case had a poor prognosis. A metastic malignancy, though mostly removed, would end up killing me just the same.

That being the case, why go for broke and try to remove every bit of the tumor when such is not a possibility anyway? That was in so many words what I asked the surgeon and very warmly he said he would keep this in mind and do his very best to effect a favorable outcome. John then thanked the surgeon and again expressed his belief that the cartilage had been at work and will alter the prognosis. "As long as I have made myself clear," was the surgeon's reply. But finally, I thought John was getting the message as he became mute and hung onto me all that evening as we prepared for the appointed hour.

* * * *

Exhausted, I retired early and fell into a profound slumber. Unbeknownst to me, a close friend came by late and asked John why he was putting me through all this – "Shouldn't nature be allowed to take its course?" she asked. When John suggested that my doctors were mistaken and that come morning they were going to be surprised, she stared at him for a minute and then quictly slipped back into the night.

Whether John got any sleep is a question. But as we left for the hour-long drive, the lonely 4 AM darkness failed to conceal his desperation. During the drive I began discussing funeral arrangements and in a fit of discomfiture John whispered, "I think it's working." I obliged by remaining silent the rest of the way.

Saturday, March 25, 1995, 5:30 AM was the appointed time, but we had arrived early. Besides having to sign papers giving my husband power of attorney to function in my behalf if critical medical decisions became necessary, there was a host of other preparations that made these early morning minutes pass quickly. And before I knew it I was on a gurney speeding toward the operating room. Having been caught up in the rush of events, I felt supremely calm and I didn't even have time to think, "This is it!" But surprisingly, I remembered one thing. John and I had recently seen a television news magazine report revealing that some anesthesiologists leave the operating room for much of the time and so I worried and asked the doctor attending me if he would remain throughout the entire operation. "Yes, I promise, I will be with you the whole time," he said. And this kind assurance was the last thing I remember before going under.

* * * *

Bone tired, my husband slumped in the waiting room and dreamily pictured the dignified surgeon skipping out and announcing, "Well, guess what? No tumor!" But it didn't happen that way. Instead, midway through the seven-hour procedure, his nurse came out and told John the brain tumor was encapsulated and probably benign. "Just relax," she said as she glided back to the operating room. And when I woke up in the intensive care room, the anathesiologist was on one side of me and John was on the other and sleepily I tried to introduce my husband to him not remembering that they had already met. The doctor then assured me that he had been with me the whole time. "That's good," I replied. "I felt safer knowing that you would be there." And soon, I would be seeing quite a number of people.

Besides my husband and a dear coworker named Hank (Henrietta) who had been keeping vigil with John in the waiting room, another coworker happened to be there with other members of her family. Her father had been injured in a sporting accident and was comatose and in the intensive care section next to mine. I guess with all the pleasantries surrounding me, it might have lightened the sterile atmosphere some. Later, my oncologist came in and gave me a big hug and expressed great satisfaction that no malignancy was apparent. A stream of others came to see me during my short hospital stay and many seemed surprised over the operation's favorable outcome. Significantly, John was no longer viewed as a little crazy – not by any of the doctors, not by any of our friends. And even I vowed to take him more seriously. John of all people was now getting respect for his apparent medical acumen!

* * * *

On Tuesday, after just three days in the hospital, I was released. Some of the nurses were worried about the early release but I was so happy to have this terrible medical burden lifted from my shoulders that I looked forward to being home with an intensity I had never experienced before and I happily acquiesced. Besides, John's "living room on wheels," the Town Car, was comfortable and had a serene ride, I reasoned. "At least you're not going home in a pickup truck," one nurse said and John and I were on our way. But talk about the best laid plans of mice and men! We were soon trapped behind an "oversize load" on the mountain pass that led home and we crept along at about five or 10 miles per hour. The pain in my neck and the back of my head became intense and there was no way to turn the car around. By making several seating adjustments, however, I finally found a position that helped, but only modestly. After a long two hours getting there, home looked better than it ever had. Happily, the pain subsided after I stretched out to rest.

The rather quiet time to follow was used not only to convalesce from the brain surgery but to ruminate on recent events and ponder their significance. During this recent hospital stay, for example, I remained off of all my "health food" supplements as per the surgeon's instructions. However, when I told the surgeon that my retching and vomiting episodes were returning because my system lacked the acidophilus I had been taking, it didn't take but a very short time for the pharmacist to appear at my bedside with acidophilus capsules. "Yes, it does help some patients settle gastrointestinal upsets," the pharmacist said. And he also agreed that it was especially important to prevent any retching or vomiting episodes because of the recent surgery.

Interestingly, I had never experienced a single serious reaction to any of the natural products I've tried. Although cautioned to stay off of the shark cartilage before and after any major surgery, it is noteworthy that I had only been off of it for a few days before the brain surgery and yet all of my blood test results were in the normal range and it was obvious that the neurosurgeon encountered no hemorrhagic problems when operating on me. In contrast to the benign effects of natural products, the side effects I suffered from chemotherapy, to give but one example, can only be described as ghastly.

Even medical tests and scans while obviously useful can also have unintended effects. My oncologist had me go in for x-rays and other tests to look for possible metastases and to check for other problems. As mentioned earlier, my gastrointestinal upsets caused by the chemotherapy had gotten so bad that he once had me go in for an an upper GI and intestinal scan using a heavy liquid called "barium" which is taken orally and its flow tracked by x-rays. As the liquid wound through my system, it was determined that I had no intestinal blockage. Yet, within days, my condition grew even worse and a second x-ray scan showed that I now had a blockage caused by the barium itself which somehow had solidified! Needless to say, I had to go through yet another treatment program to dissolve it. Thus, when I encounter medical doctors who become upset by my use of natural supplements and health foods – and I have met up with a number of them – it makes me wonder, what is going on?

Another thing we had time to consider was the brain tumor itself. It was classified as a "meningioma with no atypia" and there was no written indication that the cartilage I had been ingesting had a possible role in this unexpected outcome. By this time, we had learned that at least one bovine cartilage researcher had suggested that malignant cells may at times turn benign from the influence of cartilage therapy. We also knew that the "Swiss cheese effect" caused by shark cartilage therapy may be somewhat less apparent in some tumors. Regardless, we came to the conclusion that the medical mindset against natural supplements would have precluded an objective appraisement.

Several other factors of interest also became apparent. Only about 20 percent of the general population contracting brain cancer end up with a benign meningioma. My case was in a restricted population since I already had a metastatic cancer and, consequently, my chance of having a benign tumor was less than 20 percent, perhaps lower than five percent. That was the reason for the very dark prognosis. Yet it must be said that a possibility does exist that my brain tumor might have been completely unrelated to the ovarian cancer. It also needs to be pointed out, however, that characteristically a meningioma is encapsulated and would thus resemble a shark cartilage treated metastatic tumor.

* * * *

Despite all of his analysis and his seemingly easy acceptance of statistical probability, John had been under an enormous amount of stress and it was beginning to show. For one thing, his blood pressure was starting to spike upward erratically. Although not overly health conscious, John did keep track of his blood pressure partly because it took little effort and partly because he was very concerned about suffering a stroke. Typically, his pressure registered in the normal or near-normal range but now it was registering very high from time to time, especially on the systallic side. It wasn't necessary to convince him to go to the doctor but strangely the spikes didn't show up in the doctor's office. But as time went on John's blood pressure started to register consistently high and he was put on prescription medicine to help control it. He started taking natural substances for it as well.

The rather frequent phone conversations John had with Barney were also stressful. Regardless of any good news, Barney was becoming more and more depressed. In failing to cheer him up, John himself was leaving the phone dispirited. Fortunately, John was developing a clearer perspective on the health care industry which appeared to actually lessen his anxiety. And our mutual desperation had brought us even closer together in how we view this now unwholesome appearing world of medical politics.

* * * *

In recounting my health experiences, John uncovered many others sharing his conclusion that evidence of a vast medical-pharmaceutical cartel does exist. And it was the most highly educated people in our social circle who were the strongest in this belief. And for good reason. Supporters of a cartel obviously need to keep its true nature from being discerned by the general public. Many people have observed the behavior of the medical professionals and noted the obvious and extreme bias in favor of their own brand of health care. But fewer discern the more subtle ploys used to protect the cartel's turf and thus help ensure the continued enrichment of its members. Monopolistic aspirations infect not only commercial enterprises, to which members of the health care system belong, but as well political and religious institutions. Self-interest is simply a pervasive fact of life. But when harnessed by an appropriately free political setting, self-interest becomes more productive.

Curiously, cartels find it advantageous to generate beneficial outcomes which are widely publicized. Even illicit drug cartels commit acts of charity to soften local and even remote opposition. Its true overall cost, in both monetary and human terms, must be submerged beneath this glow to ensure survival. The portrayal of any competitor as dark and evil may enhance this luminescent cover, especially among groups proffering their high professionalism. Even upright alternative health practitioners become easy targets of this abuse because this "alternative" designation includes all that exists outside of conventional medicine, including the practice of snake handling to give but one example. Many apparently silly and otherwise questionable practices cast an easy shadow that invites attack. Some feel that by using other names such as "complementary" or "integrative" medicine, it might help shield legitimate practitioners. Actually, the opposite appears true. The more a practice or group competes with the medical profession directly, the more severe will be the latter's onslaught, agreeable sounding rubrics not withstanding. Church attendance, support groups and other social and psychological "props" are accepted, but non-pharmaceutical substances such as shark cartilage and non-conventional diagnostic practices as in chiropractic are not.

While medical cartelists brand other health care professionals as money gougers, they in effect hide the true cost of their monopolistic practices by obscuring the exchange of money. It is no secret that one hardly ever pays the doctor directly as one had in decades past. An intermediary takes the money, even if it's just a girl behind the counter. Health insurance by its very nature also obscures the connection between the high cost of health care and the system causing it. Shadow governments hide their cost to the public marvelously well by using some of their monetary gains to reward citizens from time to time. As well, their ties to "official" government bureaucracies further conceals the nature of their stealthy operations. Of course, this is essentially the case in medicine as well. For example, government sanctioned licensing not only helps protect the public but as well the licensee's profits. And the threat of losing that license is a powerful weapon to keep a constituent in line. This is no doubt why medical doctors react as though handling a hot potato when confronting a non-conventional treatment which appears to be working. The medical profession seems to be in such a state of crisis one can only wonder what would happen if a successful alternative cancer treatment became widely known. There is little doubt that medicine's biggest failing is in the treatment of chronic diseases, especially cancer. And I had noticed early on that the success I had experienced using shark cartilage was greeted with nervousness and equivocation by many in the medical field. Nevertheless, it is the high cost of medical care that is perhaps the major issue with most people.

One might notice that other professions are involved in unseemly practices. For example, anyone who bypasses the legal profession and chooses to defend himself in court is almost certain to lose. "He has a fool for a client," no matter how articulate and able, largely because he hasn't contributed to the profits of another entity which is suffering from an even greater public relations dilemma , the legal profession.

Thus, in the end what brings any cartel or monopoly to its knees is greed. In time, its costs become so prohibitive that consumers rebel and seek changes and alternatives. And this may well be what is happening in medicine today. Remember, it was a consumer reaction that spawned the HMO and added another facet to an already disturbed setting.

This, unhappily, appears to be the current state of medicine not only according to John but as well to a surprisingly large percentage of the people with whom he had spoken.

* * * *

Before my bout with ovarian cancer, John and I were but vaguely aware of Federal court decisions rebuking the American Medical Association for monopolistic practices. The destruction of the chiropractic profession, for example, had been an AMA focus for decades and, finally, in 1987 it was ordered to cease and desist by a Federal court which adjudicated this AMA effort a violation of the Sherman Antitrust Act. Why isn't this feature of the AMA more widely understood? You may want to figure out the answer to that question yourself.

The spiraling cost of biomedicine, on the other hand, was obvious. But little did we appreciate that today elderly Americans spend nearly 20 percent of their incomes on health care and this expenditure is over and above the coverage provided by Medicare and private insurance! And recent estimates that conventional medicine may soon absorb 14 percent of this Nation's gross product seem almost obscene when compared to its trifling four percent absorption of GNP in 1940.

To be sure, some expensive medical practices have been of singular benefit and people are living longer. As might be expected, however, the medical-pharmaceutical cartel often claims total credit for this enhanced longevity discounting increased individual devotion to proper diet and exercise as well as discounting the many visits to alternative practitioners which now appear to outnumber those made to conventional primary care doctors. This last comparison is especially significant because alternative costs are seldom cushioned – or veiled – by insurance programs. One reason a multimillionaire medical specialist may readily call a legitimate and far less affluent alternative practitioner a money gouger stems largely from the latter's greater dependence on open, out-of-pocket fees. "The love of money is the root of all evil" is a proverb thought hyperbolic by some observers. But is it, really?

It is generally recognized that both the best and the worst of human character is brought out and made more prominent in the presence of a crisis. Less noted, however, is that one's insights may be sharpened by the actual experience of a crisis. Thus, John's observations related to my experiences with cancer may have an unsettling starkness to them, but so be it. Both of us have changed. And anxiety stemming from the confusion and hypocrisy in the world of health care has been the key player in shaping this change.

chapter eight

It's Not Over

March, 25, 1995, the date of my brain surgery, had been permanently etched in my memory not only because of its seriousness but because I felt that a treacherous passage over a great divide had been negotiated. While not feeling home free, the conclusion held sway that my prospects could not get any worse than they had just been. Little did I know that the crystal ball I was using featured any number of cracks.

This is not to suggest any diminution of the serious close call I had. In fact, the neurosurgeon described how the fibrous overlay of the brain tumor had actually embedded itself in the skull bone due to the extreme pressure. For it to have been a benign meningioma rather than a metastatic tumor, it would had to have been growing about eight years! In the followup visits I made to see him, not once did the surgeon mention the health food supplements I was taking and, correspondingly, he spoke nary a word about the possible role the shark cartilage therapy might have played in the surgery's unexpected outcome. But the surgeon didn't appear to view us as errant "health-fooders" anymore and, furthermore, I had promptly returned to all my natural supplements except the shark cartilage. To prevent the possibility of its antiangeogenic power interfering with the surgical healing, the shark cartilage was temporarily forsaken in favor of bovine cartilage. This cartilage had also displayed anti-tumor properties but was not as promising as the shark variety. Nevertheless, John had called the leading bovine cartilage researcher and found that the bovine capsules would be safe to take following surgery.

It should be mentioned that the local naturopathic physician described earlier, while not in the foreground, was still helping us analyze events and we were seeing her on a regular basis. It was she who suggested that we telephone a West Coast shark cartilage researcher to be sure it was really necessary to forego the shark cartilage therapy following major surgery. We called and the answer was yes. (But we understand that such a restriction has since been modified).

Our pets play a significant role in our lives and wouldn't you know that the white cat that we had found 15 years ago as an abandoned and starving kitten was now suffering from feline senility and had taken a turn for the worse. Thus, just two days after coming home from the hospital, the poor cat had to be taken in and put to sleep. Just another reminder...

* * * *

My convalescence, though, was peaceful, this last reminder of death not withstanding. Having time to reflect, I suddenly remembered that in May of 1993 I did have an unusual headache that started just above the right eye and slowly progressed rearward across the right side to settle in back at the base of my skull. It was severe enough that I had brought it to the attention of my oncologist. Because it was unlike any headache I had previously experienced, he ordered a CT scan. The scan was canceled, however, after the headache disappeared and showed no signs of returning. And nearly two years later upon seeing my primary doctor about the head tremor, this strange episode had completely slipped my mind. Had I remembered and apprised him of this event, would he have had an easier time getting the MRI request through the HMO bureaucracy? Would it have made his diagnostic task easier? It was quite embarrassing just thinking about it.

Surprisingly, John had an unusual lapse of memory going forward in time. The night before my brain surgery, John had made a late telephone call to a friend of ours who is a retired nurse. She has a kindly disposition, making it easier for John to discuss his feelings, which is exactly what he did. He felt overwhelmed by all the pessimism directed his way and posed the question: Is it ever humane to give up on someone and let nature take its course? "Perhaps, but I'm sure you will know it if that time ever comes" was her thoughtful reply. This subject must have been extremely difficult for John to even broach as he had fully repressed it until this former nurse reminded him of the conversation three years later!

My convalescence from the brain surgery also provided John with some quiet time and he now seemed quite relaxed. In fact, he did something he had never done before.

Sewing and the making of clothing and other items is a hobby to which I devote considerable time. Naturally, then, I'm attracted to the instructional sewing programs on public television and would you ever guess who might for the first time sit down beside me and show an interest in my sewing? That's right, none other than my husband. The half-hour program we watched together was on quilting and how historical events had influenced some of the quilting design segments and John was so fascinated by it that he suggested "sewing may have deeper significance to it after all." Of course, I had already realized this but men can be such slow learners when it comes to the more subtle arts. But now, I had another concern.

True, I sometimes found myself caught in a tricky design problem and sometimes had called on John to render his ideas. But his sewing solutions were often so crazy that I would have given up this practice but for one thing, once in a while he would come up with a suggestion that would work and sometimes beautifully well. Yet, these happy solutions of his seemed to evolve through rank fortuity rather than any thoughtful applications of artistic talent he may possess. Thus, I couldn't help but wonder what John's sudden interest in my sewing might portend. Was I now going to receive gratuitous sewing advice? Might he actually take up sewing? This last thought seemed so ridiculous that I burst out laughing. But still, who knows?

* * * *

Although I had 30 metal staples in the back of my head holding my once severed skull bones together along with one staple decorating my right forehead (a misfire?), I suffered no nausea, no vomiting and no retching. On the whole I was feeling better than I had before the brain surgery.

The surgery was pronounced a complete success by my doctors even though the head tremors remained. For a few days following the surgery, the tremors were less pronounced. However, as I quickly regained my strength and, consequently, was up and about more, it became apparent that the surgery did little to alter the tremors. The chemotherapy must have been the culprit after all! Yet, had all this been known beforehand, the tumor's removal would still have been imperative because of the pressure it exerted and because benign tumors often continue to grow.

When John and I returned to the neurosurgeon to have my staples removed, I did mention the lone staple on my right forehead but the surgeon just laughed about it and never did tell us why it was there. But he informed us that the back portion of my brain was now covered by a newly developed man-made sheathing to help cushion it from the hard inner surface of the skull. "Until recently, *natural* sheathing taken from a cadaver would have been used," he said looking at me with just a hint of a smile. Needless to say, even without his emphasis on "natural" this revelation would have made me shiver. But the warmth of this man became all the more apparent when a little girl came skipping along just outside the open door of his office. "Did you see that young girl?" the surgeon asked. "Before I operated on her she could barely walk." Despite his outburst against my ingesting natural health foods, I couldn't help respect – and warmly like – this fine doctor who obviously took so much pride in his work. I felt myself very fortunate, indeed, to have had him as my surgeon.

* * * *

Feeling quite strong plus eager to get back to living a more normal life, I started venturing out and on April 11, 1995, John and I drove to Tucson for my blood draw. A week later, we found ourselves in my oncologist's office and the doctor was beaming. My CA-125 tumor marker had dropped to 25.1 which was in the "normal" range. He said the hormonal therapy he had me on could not have produced the positive results I had been experiencing and suggested I go off of it completely. "There is obviously something else at work here," he concluded. And happily John and I agreed and I was now off of all prescription medicine.

My oncologist did not at first speak of the cartilage but it didn't take him long to do so and to ask if I were still taking it. Of course, I answered yes but that I had now switched to the bovine cartilage temporarily because it was less likely to interfere with surgical healing. My oncologist nodded approvingly and told me to continue taking my supplements. Curiously, my oncologist never did ask me to name the traditional immune-boosting herbs, vitamins and minerals I had been taking even before I added the cartilage regimen. But John and I had the impression that he had considerable knowledge about both the shark and bovine cartilage and the only dark cloud now on the horizon came from my not feeling that well during the last few days. But I didn't think the problem serious enough to tell the doctor.

How mistaken I was as the old gastrointestinal upsets began to resurface with a vengeance. From experience, I knew that the ingestion of the acidophilus had helped significantly as had the back massages administered by my husband, but now these standbys seemed to help less. The suffering I endured April 25 through 28 was especially intense and I wondered if an important trip we were planning might be impossible to take.

My niece, Kerria, was scheduled to graduate from the University of Evansville in Indiana on May 6, 1995, and I did want to be there. But my gastrointestinal rumblings were at their worst when John and I went to see the neurosurgeon for my follow-up visit April 27. The neurosurgeon sensed I had something on my mind and so I told him about my desire to make this 3,700-mile round trip expecting a resounding "No." To our surprise he seemed to favor the idea suggesting we avoid air travel and thus it's variations in air pressure. "Otherwise, if the trip is important to you I see no reason why you shouldn't go as long as you take it easy and get plenty of rest," he said.

Buoyed by the surgeon's sanguine suggestion, we made ready and left that Sunday, April 30. After a very shaky start that nearly caused us to turn back, the trip went rather smoothly. As expected, I suffered from nausea and burning sensations in the esophagus but little else except for the first two days when I had the full range of upsets and was very sick, indeed. Although I was only eating about one-third of normal and was obviously losing weight, I managed a rather busy schedule once there. With so many of my relations to see both at the graduation and in our home state of Illinois, it took John's considerable effort to get me to slow down and set aside time to rest. During all of our travel, though, I made sure that I did plenty of vigorous walking to help prevent another blood clot from forming in my left leg.

During our return, John devised a plan that he concluded would make the travel time pass more easily for me. He divided the return journey into short, predetermined segments. For example, he might say, "OK, we'll stop and take a break at the town 80 miles ahead," and, indeed, this procedure helped considerably because it took my mind off of the many miles we had to travel. Although John did all of the driving, he still had an easy time since we covered but about 350 miles per day. It was back in 1971 when we last made this trip by automobile and the intervening 24 years produced a population explosion, especially in Arizona and parts of Illinois, which was strikingly evident – and shocking! Obviously, population growth can have a flip side.

During the first five days following our return home, I felt reasonably well. In fact, my blood draw of May 16 while only revealing a slightly lower CA-125 tumor marker of 23.6, helped buoy my spirits considerably. Also, my rheumatoid arthritis symptoms were held in check and John and I surmised that the bovine cartilage might very well be helping although we guessed that the effects of the shark cartilage were still in play and probably would continue their residual role for months to come. But my gastrointestinal tremors started to worsen again and in looking back I wondered how I made it through the nearly 4,000-mile trip so smoothly.

As explained earlier, I was receiving Shiatzu finger pressure treatments and these helped some. But on May 27, one treatment, by focusing primarily on the esophagus and stomach, gave me solid temporary relief in the form of a restful nap very soon afterward and an usually sound sleep that night. But on balance, my condition was trending downward and although my weight varied some from week to week it too reflected this trend and by June 1, 1995, my weight was down some 25 pounds from normal, standing at 132.

Alarmed as my weight continued inexorably downward, I attempted to eat very small meals but have them more often. Yet, even this approach failed to reverse the weight slide. My internist had encouraged me to drink Ensure as a supplement and not to worry about eating fattening foods. But by June 7, I was having so much gastrointestinal pain that by night I was unable to sleep and by day I was feeling completely drained and barely able to function.

Although my naturopathic physician prescribed gastric enzymes which did reduce the burning in the lower esophagus, they failed to moderate the two bottlenecks I often sensed after eating. It felt as though my system had two gates, one at the bottom of the esophagus and a second in the stomach. Seemingly, if the food managed to pass through the first gate, it might be blocked by the second and, of course, closure at either point would result in my feeling full and nauseated.

Interestingly, resting or sleeping on my right side seemed to lessen my discomfort and I was to later learn the reason: lying on the left side puts greater pressure on the internal organs. But for reasons not in the least understood, holding a pillow rather tightly against my stomach while at rest also eased the pain. The aftermath of the chemotherapy presented any number of mysteries, not the least of which was why during this period of incessant torment did my blood draw of June 13 reveal a CA-125 tumor marker of only 13.1 (down from 23.6), a very fortunate development, indeed! But it would be Thursday June 22, 1995, that would witness a sad passage.

On this warm, bright Thursday we were in Tucson attending an informational meeting sponsored by an HMO and on the way home I became desperately ill and for the first time since contracting ovarian cancer I threw up in the car. At home, I vomited twice more and gloom seemed to enshroud me as I fell into a fitful sleep.

The following morning I awoke pain free yet as I stood up I found myself weak and trembling. In weighing myself, I was now down to 128 pounds. But soon I felt stronger and somehow I felt that my prospects would ultimately brighten.

* * * *

Barney, on the other hand, because of his deepening depression had become impossible to cheer up and was becoming less communicative even when he was the one initiating the telephone call. He had actually been doing quite well on the cartilage by any reasonable measure, but simply could not stand the uncertainty surrounding his condition and now he had fallen on the hospital steps and broken his leg. John pointed out how lucky he was to have fallen so close to medical help but Barney didn't see it that way. To him it was the damnedest luck to have fallen in the first place. He had daily nursing help provided by a New York State agency and, in fact, John had talked to the nurse and she spoke optimistically of Barney being "up and around in no time." But this was not to be.

Not having heard from Barney in some time, John rang his apartment but no one answered. John then telephoned Barney's friend for information, and the news was bad. Barney had died from apparent suicide.

Authorities had told the friend that Barney's death was not caused by the cancer. In fact, the friend was aware of Barney's apparent success in keeping the cancer under control and was interested in learning more about cartilage therapy in the event he ever contracted cancer. John was on the phone for perhaps half an hour trying to answer all his questions.

The friend said that Barney was the quintessential loner with no relatives nearby and very few friends and that Barney did not seem to be the type who would call all over the world looking for a cancer cure.

Of course John wanted to know the date of death. It was that warm, trouble-plagued Thursday, June 22, 1995.

chapter nine

The Chemo Fallout Continues

Outside of his intractable pessimism, Barney's prospects had every appearance of being more favorable than mine. For example, he told us that his chemotherapy treatments didn't bother him that much, that they simply didn't work as his metastatic colon cancer continued to grow and spread. Upon being pronounced terminal with only a year to live, he sidestepped his doctors and investigated alternative treatments and appeared to have done so without outside help or support. He was alone and acted alone and John and I realized even at this rather early stage in my own battle against cancer that such solitary initiative was remarkable. There was something deep and enduring in this man and John at first was bewildered as to what went wrong.

One thing was obvious, John and Barney didn't share feelings or personal experiences but approached this life-threatening disease of cancer in a cold, clinical manner. There was not that much given over to "fluff" as John would say. Barney had actually experienced success: his osteoarthritis of the knees had disappeared soon after starting the cartilage therapy; his CEA tumor marker had gone down dramatically and the bounce it took may have well been just that, a bounce, and if not, the subsequent chemo he had did appear to work where it hadn't previously; and, finally, it appeared as though he could have ultimately gotten on with his life experiencing but few restraints. The uncertainty surrounding Barney's cancer may well have been overwhelming for him, but why? John had somewhat offhandedly suggested to Barney that he might find a support group helpful but he declined the suggestion. And after reflecting on this and other events, John finally concluded that no man can be an island unto himself. Of course I knew this all along but John's conversion to this proposition altered his thinking about the course I should follow as I faced the battle of my life. He was now encouraging me to investigate support groups I might wish to attend.

* * * *

Just three days following Barney's death, I needed all the support John and my doctors could provide as I developed a severe pain deep in the middle of my chest. Actually, at times the pain seemed to emanate from just within my back. And nothing would relieve it – not standing; not sitting; not lying down; not deep breathing; not walking; not John's massage. There was no shortage of breath nor branching out of the pain so it didn't appear to be a heart attack but I did fear a retching episode and thus for some time I took nothing. Finally, I quickly swallowed two Tylenol tablets with water and paused to see if they would stay down. They did and within an hour the pain subsided.

John had been in contact with my doctor's office and he wanted to rush me to the emergency room. But I didn't want to go because I had been experiencing other strange pains and they would in time disappear never to return. Nevertheless, I was in my internist's office the next morning and my doctor immediately scheduled another upper GI scan. He also put me on ulcer medication.

The upper GI barium scan revealed inflammation of the lower intestinal tract and a very long "passage time" as it took the barium about five hours to wind through my system. The radiologist seemed concerned that the cause of my problem could be the cancer. On the brighter side, the ulcer medicine (Carafate) I had started was apparently calming my gastrointestinal upsets.

More good days allowed me to walk more to help keep my left leg clear of clots and help improve my digestion. But on balance, my condition hadn't improved that much and, unfortunately, I still had plenty of bad days. Thus, when my blood draw of July 11, 1995, exhibited a CA-125 marker of 11.3 it really came as a surprise for several reasons. First, the marker number without the decimal fraction corresponded with the 11th day of July when the blood sample was taken. And, similarly, you'll remember, the June marker of 13.1 matched the 13th day of that month. Then, too, John found the date of Barney's death, June 22, 1995, rather meticulously etched in a hard steel support found in one of the clinic restrooms. Needless to say, John and I are not in the least superstitious, but still there are those who might attach some meaning to it.

What we were more concerned about, really, was that my tumor markers had been in the normal range for some months now and these favorable counts didn't accompany any significant improvements in my physical condition which in some ways had actually grown worse. It was fortunate that my internist, especially, kept reminding us that the strange torments I now suffered could all be accounted for by the chemotherapy I had endured so many months before. Otherwise, at this stage, we might have concluded that the CA-125 tumor marker assay had gone haywire and that my malignancy was surreptitiously raging out of control and that the cartilage was not working. As it was, we were beginning to wonder if the bovine cartilage was working better than we had expected. But my intuition told me that it was the residual effects of the shark cartilage that was carrying the yeoman load. John, the realist, wasn't so sure but I couldn't argue the point because everything about this disease of mine seemed essentially unpredictable.

* * * *

Backed by John's renewed encouragement, I started investigating some of the support groups connected to my nonprofit HMO and uncovered two I thought appropriate. The first was a general support group for practically anyone. It didn't matter what kind of cancer a person had and spouses could be included. So I talked

John into attending a session with me but he became noticeably bored by some of the subjects brought up and I could see he was not the support group type. Thus, I ended up going to a gynecological group that excluded husbands (and other males) and found it more promising. I think John actually preferred reading in an adjacent hallway seating area as from the start he didn't seemed to mind waiting.

The GYN group met weekly on Tuesdays at 3 PM and following a short period of sporatic attendance I made up my mind to become a regular participant. And I soon realized that it was very comforting associating with women whose experiences sometimes matched my own and my horizons also began to expand as the warm communion with other group members fostered in me an enhanced feeling of kinship with cancer patients in general. On the practical side, John and I had to go to the City of Tucson anyway on a regular basis for shopping, and driving there each Tuesday and capping the day at the support session evolved into a pleasant routine. Then, too, the women of this particular assemblage had a well-deserved reputation for warmth and helpfulness.

It didn't take long before I developed some very close friends within the group and the exchanges we had were often exhilarating and fun. But John who almost always found himself alone became the object of considerable notice particularly from volunteers and other women who walked by. The participants in my group had also earned the reputation for being nonstop talkers and the support sessions often ran late and John, the dutiful husband, would quietly sit and read or, at times, look up at the ceiling. It didn't take long for many of the passersby to smile and comment on his high sense of duty and on the talkativeness of the distaff side. The other husbands didn't have to be concerned as they lived nearby and could run errands or have their wives drive themselves to the sessions. So John most often sat alone to absorb and reflect on the high spirited teasing directed his way. And upon the group's ending, he sometimes acted as though I had come to the rescue.

* * * *

Despite the happy support sessions, the latter part of July didn't see any real improvement in my physical condition as a series of strange pains came and went. Not only did these stabbing pains affect my abdomen and upper body, but now my hips were involved especially the right one. Although I continued to have an underlying unwell feeling, I did experience one relief, however, for the vomiting and retching took an unexpected hiatus. And another kind of relief soon followed.

My internist seemed somewhat perplexed by all my physical torments and had me undergo another onocostint scan during the first days of August. And the x-ray films showed no "lights" suggesting an absence of cancer cells. Of course, I was much relieved over this news but my doctor appeared less so. It was only later that my internist explained that a second scan might not be as reliable as the first since the body's immune system has already been exposed to the protein "carriers" of radioactive material and now upon recognizing them as foreign be fully mobilized to destroy them. One might remember that these proteins normally bypass normal cells and attach themselves to malignant ones. Of course, it is the radioactive material carried by the proteins that is revealed by the onocostint x-ray scan.

On Sunday, August 5, 1995, I started retching and vomiting again ending a glorious 20-day respite. Additionally, late that night a pain developed in my chest that by the next morning became so severe I nearly passed out. John called my internist's emergency number and was told by the doctor on duty to come immediately to the emergency room. As we drove to the Tucson Medical Center, the pain became so debilitating that upon arrival I could barely move and was wheeled into ER. A nurse took me aside and asked me to rate the severity of the pain from one to 10, the highest number being the greatest pain ever experienced. I rated it 10. Although I had been having less severe pains all along both in the chest and other areas, the doctor, naturally, wanted to eliminate the possibility I was having a heart attack. And that possibility was promptly eliminated as the test results were negative.

Because my intense pain could have been caused by the passing of gallstones, I soon found myself on the operating table undergoing a small incision for a laparoscopic examination and removal of my gallbladder. But the surgeon was confronted with a pancreas so inflamed that he had to close the incision having only probed my abdominal cavity. And what he saw was all the more disturbing because my organs "were bound together as though covered by super glue." He also said that once the infection was brought under control using antibiotics, "a full-cut gallbladder removal would be necessary" and that he didn't look forward to doing the operation "as the surgeon doing it will confront some difficult problems." Although he informed me that the pancreatic infection could have been fatal and that I was very fortunate to have had it discovered in time, he did save the very best news for last: his probe uncovered no cancer.

A little later a laboratory analysis of my abdominal serum also revealed an absence of malignancy which was a needed lift as my hospital stay promised to be a long one. Besides the administration of antibiotics through an IV, liquid nourishment was similarly infused. Later, I was weaned to solid, low-fat foods and was allowed to resume taking the bovine cartilage that I had now been off of for seven days. Although the surgeon didn't seem privy to my cartilage therapy, the other doctors – as well as some of the nurses – asked about it and encouraged me to continue taking it sometimes adding that "it can't do any harm." After an eight-day stay, I was finally released from the hospital the 14th of August.

* * * *

Because unexpected events seemed to fly by me so wildly, my return from the hospital seemed very much like a happy landing as it gave me time to repose in quiet reflection. And what reflections they were! So far I was surviving and I was becoming alert to the fact that my will to live played such a pivotal role that I must not let my guard down not even for a second and remain fully atop my condition.

It was hard, though, because the mysteries involved in my illness were so unsettling – not only for me but for my doctors as well – and they weren't getting any easier to unravel. For example, my naturopathic physician had explained why John's massages were so soothing and relieved my pains. She had said muscular spasm respond very readily to massage, but now I was developing muscle pains that didn't respond to massage that much and for this there appeared to be no ready explanation save a somewhat nebulous one, nerve and organ damage caused by the chemotherapy. Could the nerve damage stop my heart? Are some of my organs beyond repair? These and other questions were coming to mind, yet I knew I had to look forward and cultivate hope.

And, indeed, forward my sights were aimed as I wanted to attend an alternative medical convention sponsored by the Cancer Control Society to be held over this 1995 Labor Day weekend in Pasadena, California. Although the conference itself lasted just the three days of the holiday weekend, the nonprofit Society on subsequent days sponsored a doctor's symposium plus bus excursions into neighboring Mexico to visit eight cancer treatment clinics. These clinics employ mostly nontoxic natural treatment protocols many of which would be disallowed in the United States. Of course, I knew my physical condition precluded taking in but a portion of the very extensive program offered but I still had a fierce desire to attend.

Since I had just been released from the hospital in the middle of August in less than stable condition, John suggested we confer first with my surgeon, fully expecting that he would recommend against my taking the trip. And – surprise – despite my continued weight loss and sporatic pains, the doctor suggested that if the conference was important to us to go ahead and make the trip. Which is exactly what we did.

* * * *

The 550-mile, day-long drive was essentially uneventful as I held up better than expected. Because the convention brought together in one place many health authorities from around the world, I felt that it would be highly informative, and I was not disappointed. In fact, it was an eye opener! There were so many treatment options and combinations thereof presented that it was difficult keeping up with them all.

Although each speaker was usually limited to only a half-hour, the presentations began as early as 8 AM and ended as late as 11 PM! It was obvious that the large, 500-plus seating of the Pasadena Hilton Ballroom accommodated many health professionals some of whom appeared to receive educational or promotional credit for attending. Medical doctors, naturopathic physicians, nutritionists, chiropractors, a dentist, and even a veterinarian turned people doctor were on hand as speakers as were once terminal cancer patients available to tell their stories of survival. The atmosphere seemed electric with anticipation unlike past conventional conferences we had attended in Tucson which tended to be stodgy and poorly attended.

At the Cancer Control Society convention we were immediately struck by the great number of health product exhibits and booths which almost overflowed the immediate foyer and created a bit of a commercial atmosphere. Had we attended more of the conventional health conferences we might have become fully accustomed to the plodding and colorless environment so often associated with them and thus would have found this new atmosphere a bit like a carnival as well. As it was, conversing with these alternative health enthusiasts was revealing as so many of them were attracted to this field because of their own experiences in surviving cancer. John and I realized that because of my survival so far, we were now a part of this group.

To be sure, some appeared to be offering more hope than cure, more snake oil than substance but at the same time it doesn't take that much acumen to sort out the more questionable claims. Still, the uncertainty inherent in a free market atmosphere is too much for some people and perhaps this is part of the reason that the majority of those drawn here beyond the medico-pharmaceutical cartel are frequently above average in both education and income, as shown by numerous surveys. Interestingly, we met one young man who was studying to be a naturopathic doctor who nodded approvingly of our approach in fighting my cancer. "A person has to be able and willing to do the extensive homework necessary," he said. "Otherwise, the choices made are likely to be based only on emotion and hope." Of course, we were painfully aware of how supremely difficult this investigatory process could be.

During one intermission, John and I narrowly avoided bumping into Dr. I. William Lane, co-author of the book, *Sharks Don't Get Cancer*. He was hobbling into the conference room on crutches, one foot enlarged by copious bandaging. He had injured his foot overseas while working to help other countries establish clinical trials using shark cartilage therapy. A short man but with a giant voice and energized persona, he was quick to let me know how thoroughly pleased he was that my cartilage therapy had worked and tweaked my cheek for emphasis only adding how sorry he was that it didn't work for everyone.

Lane's presentation that Sunday midday was warmly received and we could hear some in the audience conversing aloud about the favorable results they or a friend had had in using it. Following the presentation, survey forms were distributed asking those who had employed shark cartilage therapy to answer a series of questions. In response to one question, I had answered, "The cartilage therapy saved my life." Little did I realize that filling out this form would some months later nearly land me on a Fox Television talk show. (However, I had a second and more dangerous blood clot in my left leg again and was unable to make the trip to California to participate on the show.)

The three-day conference featured more than 40 presenters

some with recognizable names, such as: Charlotte Gerson, daughter of Max Gerson, M.D., and President of the Gerson Institute through which she continues to promote her renowned father's nutrition-based treatment protocol for cancer; Earl Mindell, R.Ph., Ph.D., pharmacist and nutritionist and author of *Vitamin Bible*, a best seller; Patrick Quillin, Ph.D., R.D., Registered Dietitian and author of *Beating Cancer With Nutrition*; Douglas Brodie, M.D., granted the right to treat his patients with Metabolic Therapy by the Superior Court of Auburn, California, in a landmark case for freedom; and, as already mentioned, I. William Lane, Ph.D. And the conference topics seemed to cover almost the full range of alternative cancer treatments. However, despite all this going on, the outside media seemed to narrow its focus on one young man who was scheduled to appear on the Sunday afternoon segment set aside to hear two-minute presentations mostly from once terminal cancer patients who had managed to recover using alternative therapies.

The young man in the media spotlight was now 17-year-old Billy Best who had contracted a lymphatic cancer and had gained national attention by running away from home to avoid the chemotherapy he found so debilitating. Upon returning home, his parents, William and Susan Best, agreed to allow their son to try an alternative approach to see if that would work before resorting to chemotherapy. A substance largely made up of camphor and nitrogen called 714X was used along with an herbal brew call Essiac. And this regimen coupled with a largely vegetarian diet appeared to bring about a remission and now Billy was scrambling to get into line with a large number of other people to give his two-minute presentation.

As the first person looked up to speak, many of the media gazed back at her and showed some impatience as Billy Best had somehow ended up in the middle of the procession. She managed to get past the media yawns and other displays of indifference and deliver an effective presentation, and so did those who followed.

Everyone, including members of the media, came to pay rapt attention as the moving stories progressed. Billy Best told his poignant story and although the media representatives seemed satisfied, some stayed on to hear from still others. John and I realized why this segment of the program seemed so popular: it showed that terminal patients, indeed, had alternatives and that these not only offered hope but frequently extended life as well. John suggested I would be up there speaking next year. Yes, if I live that long, was my thought.

Indeed, John and I were impressed by both the depth and scope of the program and although the Cancer Control Society bills itself as an "educational, charitable and scientific Society supported by contributions and memberships," it was more.

Time had been set aside on the program to consider the politics of cancer and from the discussions engendered it became obvious that the organization also exercised an important civil rights function, especially for terminal cancer patients. As had been mentioned, John in researching alternatives for me sensed almost immediately that little freedom prevailed in this country's health arena. And now, upon hearing how doctors outside of the pharmaceutical cartel were being harassed, having their licenses to practice threatened, even having to face possible prison time, it became apparent to us there was work that needed to be done.

Although this country's constitution implicitly guarantees such medical freedom by the broad sweep of its pronouncements, it does not precisely enumerate it, allowing the powerful cartel interests to effectively sully and crush this most basic freedom. And some of our founding fathers worried about not taking the time to be more specific about this matter and, of course, their fears have been justified.

chapter ten

A Missed Wedding

Even though I had few gastrointestinal upsets while attending the Cancer Control Society convention, fatigue did frequently overtake me and so John and I only attended the three-day conference itself. To be sure, we especially wanted to take the tour of the cancer treatment centers in Mexico but we realized that it would put too much strain on me. As it was, I had to choose which conference presentations I most wanted to attend and seek out comfortable chairs in the outer lobby and catnap through those which appeared less promising. Of course, John had more energy and attended more of these sessions. He also spent considerable time during the intermissions talking to the numerous health care practitioners and cancer researchers present.

During the entire sojourn, I had continued my walking exercises especially after eating and perhaps this was one reason why the return trip home was so happily routine. But on September 8, I was back at the Tucson cancer clinic for blood draws in preparation for the full-cut gallbladder surgery mentioned earlier. My weight was now down to a worrisome 122 pounds and my CA-125 tumor marker had risen from 11.3 to 27.5 and my doctors seemed unworried by this rise attributing it to the stresses I had encountered in the past two months. But for more than five months I had not been able to take the shark cartilage because of the surgeries and I felt it was payoff time. But despite my misgivings, John agreed with the doctors.

And on September 12, the same surgeon who earlier had laparoscopically uncovered the "super glue" adhesions, now had little trouble removing my gallbladder and found only "ribbons of cholesterol" in place of the expected gallstones. But more important, the surgeon was surprised to find no cancer cells present and it thus suggested that my other doctors and John were right about the tumor marker rise. The surgeon explained that any gallstones I may have had had already passed through my system and caused the pain that I had found so excruciating weeks earlier and it apparently had nothing to do with the cancer. But even this assurance didn't allay my suspicion that the ovarian cancer was on its way back.

* * * *

After being released from the hospital September 14, my digestive problems leveled off somewhat, but I continued to lose weight and I was looking skeletal. Even though I was drinking lots of Ensure, "complete, balanced nutrition," as directed by my doctors, I was still a bit shaky and weak. Nevertheless, I was buoyed by the prospect of attending the October 7 wedding of my niece, Susan, in Houston, Texas as I fully expected to go. But John had been very carefully checking my daily calorie intake and found it insufficient to maintain even the reduced weight level of 119 pounds I had now dropped to and was voicing his concern that I was going downhill fast. I told him we were going to the wedding.

I need not have to tell you how I ended up in my internist's office Friday, September 29, about a week before the scheduled ceremony and just days before our planned departure. Yet John was not the only one noticing just how frail I was as people were beginning to openly stare at me and now my doctor seemed concerned. He examined me thoroughly and gave his OK to take the trip. However, he scheduled an upper GI scan for me the following Monday the results of which he said could be discussed with us upon our return from Houston.

We were packed and ready to leave the following Tuesday, but when we arrived home Monday afternoon following the scan, my internist's voice on our answering machine sounded urgent and I was told to immediately call his office, which I did. He quickly came to the phone and told me the scan results were alarming. My stomach was now double its normal size and the upper intestines were also greatly distended. "You can't take your trip, he said. "You must undergo surgery immediately."

Although I was greatly shocked, I still managed to question whether it couldn't wait until after the planned trip, but my doctor firmly disabused me of the notion saying that I would end up in a hospital elsewhere if we were to venture away. As it was, I was checked into our local Tucson Medical Center hospital by 8 AM Tuesday, October 3, 1995, the time we had planned to depart for Houston, and I hardly had time to cry.

* * * *

My primary care internist had already summoned one of my HMO's surgeons to meet me at the hospital and I remained dressed in a loose fitting outfit that tended to hide my bony appearance. This coupled with the make-up I wore gave me a rather robust appearance. The young surgeon appeared at the door just as a nurse whom I had already gotten well acquainted with from so many other visits had joked about how much I must like the hospital. We were both bent over in laughter when the surgeon stared at me and asked, "What is wrong with you?" Completely bewildered by our continued laughter, he blurted out, "You look fine to me."

The nurse left and I tried to explain to the surgeon that I had a happy disposition and I often acted this way whether sick or well. But the surgeon had not been able to find my records and suggested surgery might not be necessary owing to the vibrant condition I seemed to be in. Of course my countenance brightened as we were still packed for my niece's wedding. But my internist had just stepped in and was obviously disturbed by what he was hearing.

Within minutes, the now rather flustered surgeon was under a barrage of questions from my internist primarily about having not located my records. The young surgeon was signaled out to the hallway by my internist to continue their discussion and in about five minutes my primary care internist returned and said the surgery to free up my digestive organs was on for that night.

My internist then beckoned John to come with him. As they slowly walked down the hallway, John was told that delaying the surgery would result in a further loss of weight and might well erase any hopes of recovery and that it had to be done immediately. Of course, John agreed wholeheartedly. (My internist later told us that this operation was quite a gamble because such adhesions often grow right back again).

Soon I was dressed in hospital garb and being wheeled to the radiology department for more x-rays in preparation for the surgery. While waiting my turn, the young surgeon stepped in and solemnly explained that he had found my records and that doing the surgery was indeed critical. The surgery would be far from easy, he said, and he might have to do a colostomy wherein the solid wastes are shunted to a bag. "Only do it if it's a life-or-death matter," was my immediate response. And the young surgeon became even more solemn suggesting that a metastatic malignancy might well be causing the problem but that he would do his very best.

As if I didn't have enough to worry about upon being returned to my room, the nurses were waiting to insert the surgical IV in my arm and I knew from past experience that it wasn't going to be easy. In fact, the procedure took an inordinate amount of time and was more painful than it had ever been because my already much punctured arm veins were in an implacable state and simply collapsed with just a touch of the needle. But the procedure was finally accomplished and I was allowed to rest, but only briefly.

The nurses returned to insert a NG (nasogastric tube) which

is a catheter that is inserted up the nose and then down the throat and into the stomach. It can be used to administer supplemental nutrients or in my case to pump out gastric juices. The nurses first measured the length of tubing necessary and then had me sip water through a straw and keep swallowing until the tube was thus drawn into the stomach. Haste was necessary because I was scheduled for surgery at 7 PM. But as they approached the final step, attaching the catheter to the pump, we were informed that my operation would have to be canceled because of emergency surgery resulting from a bad automobile accident. The catheter, however, was to remain in place throughout most of my hospital stay.

* * * *

The older surgeon who had discovered my "super glue" adhesions and just recently removed my gallbladder had been out of town. Now, the following morning very early, he was at my bedside gently nudging my shoulder and calling my name to talk to me about scheduling the surgery for that day. He discussed the seriousness of it and that there might be no choice but to do a colostomy. In turn, I asked him to perform the operation since he already knew what to expect. Although he let me know that the younger surgeon was fully up to the task, he agreed to do the surgery and said it would have to be scheduled for sometime that evening. Again, I voiced my aversion to the colostomy and although this surgeon was usually hurried and laconic he did take the time to listen to me and responded sympathetically.

The chalkboard at the nurse's station had me scheduled for an afternoon surgery with the younger doctor and I kept making inquiries about it during the morning and early afternoon telling the nurses and anyone else who would listen that the older surgeon had promised to do it and it was supposed to be scheduled for later.

About 3 PM, the chalkboard still showed no change and a new nurse on duty stepped out to investigate why. While she was out investigating, an attendant came in with a gurney to take me to presurgery and I had to tell him that there was a problem and that there would be a delay. Meanwhile, my internist called me and I explained the problem to him and just as I hung up the nurse returned. She, too, was sympathetic saying that it was my body involved and, therefore, my right to refuse the surgery until an understanding was reached.

By this time I had quite an audience: several nurses, the bewildered attendant as well as my husband who had arrived some time earlier. Within minutes, the older surgeon telephoned me inquiring about the problem and I reminded him that he had promised to do the surgery. I could feel my audience listening intently as I used the same teaching strategies I had evolved over my many years of teaching young children to convince the surgeon that he should keep his promise.

Apparently, he had heard enough and promised that both of them would do the surgery but that it would have to be scheduled later. Feeling much relieved, I agreed and, finally, the astonished gurney attendant was dismissed by the amused nurses.

* * * *

When I was wheeled into the presurgery room at about 7 PM, the older surgeon greeted me with a broad smile and remarked that the telephone conversion reminded him of his own primary school days and being scolded by the teacher. After performing a short examination and finding me fit for surgery, he assured me during a lighthearted exchange that he would be there in the operating room. And, as if on cue, the younger surgeon came in and also seemed amused and assured me that the two of them would work together for the most favorable outcome possible. As I was being wheeled into the sterile and cool operating room, I realized I was actually taking control of my medical care and depending less on John. And it was a warm and satisfying feeling.

But poor John, indeed, had considerable waiting to do as the operating time extended well beyond the hour-and-a-half estimate and it wasn't until close to 11 PM that the older surgeon came out and told him that my organs had been cut free and no cancer was found. With his usual briskness, he told John that his partner was finishing up and would soon be out to explain everything in detail. And in about 15 minutes the young surgeon did come out and clearly had much to tell.

The surgery had taken so long because no cancer was evident and much time had been spent exploring the entire abdominal cavity to make sure any malignancy hadn't been missed. "I searched and searched but there is no cancer," he emphasized to John while speaking as though someone had told him that the malignancy had to be there someplace. The young surgeon even demonstrated with his hands some of the exploratory maneuvers he used in his failed quest. Then leaning back and shaking his head back and forth ever so slightly, he suggested that it was a good thing the chemotherapy was effective because it left a thick fibroid overlay that severely bound the abdominal organs together. After John told him that it wasn't the chemotherapy but rather shark cartilage that had actually worked, the young surgeon's facial expression turned blank and he volunteered no response. But he had more on his mind.

For one thing, the surgeon observed no peristalsis of my small intestines. This coupled with no specific blockage being uncovered suggested a possible neurological dysfunction. But because no discrete blockage was found, he was simply bereft of a solid explanation as to why my stomach and upper intestinal tract was so enlarged.

* * * *

My subsequent days in the hospital seemed to revolve around the stomach pump. It was on almost continuously, and periodically the amount of stomach secretions pumped out would be measured. All but one of these measures showed excessive gastric secretions. But the nurses seemed pleased by the gurgling and other noises my stomach made from time to time, indicating my gastrointestinal system was functioning, at least on a limited basis. But I was not allowed to eat anything but a few ice chips and was given a full nutritional substance (TPN) intravenously.

One day I was given barium sulfate to run through my digestive system so that another upper GI scan could be taken. Even though I had to be given morphine to calm painful muscle spasms that developed on my left side, the scan was finally completed and happily no blockage was revealed. Then the nurses made sure I was given some mineral oil and milk of magnesia to avoid another barium blockage. The older surgeon had written an order for a second dose but I was now suffering from diarrhea and suggested the extra dose was unnecessary and the surgeon rescinded the order. Eventually I began to feel very hungry.

No matter how hungry I felt, the nurse said no food consumption could be allowed. However, an attendant overheard my request and suggested a popsicle might be permitted since it was just flavored ice anyway. The nurse agreed, and asked with just a slight twist of drama about my flavor preference. "Cherry" said I, and I savored the popsicle as long as I could and it truly was the most delicious I had ever had.

More delights were to follow as the nurses and I could watch the cherry fluid pass through the catheter and swirl to a colorful rest in the collection jar. One nurse remarked how someone walking in without knowing about my cherry flavored popsicle could view the highly colored collection jar with alarm.

At 4 AM Sunday, October 15, I was awakened to have my catheter and intravenous tubing removed and though this was a great relief, John and I had sensed from the nurses' facial expressions and the rather dark exchanges between them that not all had gone that favorably. Yet, they tried me on some liquids for a day followed by a very limited amount of solid food to see what would happen.

It was obvious by all of the visits I had from the hospital staff and my doctors that I was under rather intense observation and I had the feeling that if this eating trial failed it would mean a return to the stomach pump and intravenous feeding. But surprise was registered by one and all as I managed to keep down the tiny portions of solid food such as blueberry crepes and did not become sick. But preparations for my departure from the hospital became bittersweet.

Although the nonprofit Tucson Medical Center is a sprawling single story structure in which the units are spread out even more by numerous (and beautiful) outdoor patios and other open spaces, a closeness among staff members seemed to exist. And I felt such a warm regard for many of those of my unit that I was nearly reduced to tears as I started gathering my things to leave. Even the nurses and others going off shift would stop by and give me a big and sometimes tearful hug.

John was with me during much of this time and had observed, as had I, that some of the more experienced staff members seemed powerless not to express subtle cues about my very dismal prospects. And only hours before I was to be released from the hospital on Tuesday, October 17, my 14th day and the longest stint for me ever, John was on the hospital phone talking to my naturopathic physician and pouring out all his worry. But she had not given up on me and had a plan.

chapter eleven

Mind Power

The hospital release did not accompany any apparent improvement in my condition since my gastrointestinal distress, though less severe, did continue to suppress my appetite and my weight continued slowly downward. Surprisingly, my weight had stabilized while in the hospital eating little or nothing and being nourished intravenously, yet now it didn't take but a day or two to realize that very little improvement in my appetite was apparent. Also, John had no idea on what to do next.

My naturopathic doctor suggested to him that I receive treatments from a hypnotherapist. Stunned, John countered with a long silence. "You should remember, John, that Kay doesn't think the way you do," the doctor said, no doubt realizing that this was the understatement of the millennium. "Kay has been through so much and I think the hypnotic treatments would be a natural extension of the support group sessions she has found so beneficial." John realized that the support meetings of the past several months had given me comfort and hope and thus acceded to the idea noting that he hadn't even entertained the notion of hypnotherapy.

Regardless, the arrangements were made and at 9 AM, Tuesday, just one week following my release from the hospital, John and I were seated at a small table facing a kindly man who appeared braced for a storm promising thunder and very high winds. As I calmly fleshed out the sketchy outline he had been given concerning my case, the psychologist soon relaxed and began asking me numerous questions. He was trying to determine whether to use a direct approach and immediately target the appetite problem or delve more deeply into my psyche. But John jumped in and settled the question.

He told the therapist that I had actually taken all this in remarkable stride and had no hint of a deep-rooted emotional problem and suggested concentrating on the eating problem itself. The psychologist agreed and remarked on how calm and collected I was during this first session and that he had essentially concluded the same thing. His hope was to restore a positive attitude to my eating and thereby soothe and help energize my gastrointestinal organs to function more normally. Now I understood why he called his approach "behavioral medicine."

Middle-aged and supremely calm and confident, the therapist came highly recommended by several medical practitioners and I was immediately impressed by his sincerity and by the intensity of his efforts to help me. Because he had a Ph.D., everyone addressed him as "Doctor" and the title fit so admirably not only because of his competence as a therapist but also his interest in, and knowledge of, almost any underlying medical problem a patient might have. In fact, I soon learned that his wife had a rare and terminal autoimmune condition and he was investigating possible alternative treatments for her.

My apparent success with shark cartilage not only in controlling my ovarian cancer but as well my rheumatoid arthritis, a disease also having autoimmune roots, encouraged my therapist to start his own investigation of cartilage therapy. And it didn't take long for him to inquire about what I might know concerning its potential to ease his wife's condition. John's focus, however, had been almost entirely on my cancer and we had no idea. But being investigatory himself, it did appear that if there was something out there that held promise, the therapist would likely uncover it.

Needless to say, I felt very much at ease with this very special and warm person and under his tutelage I began feeling more serene. Even when my blood draw of October 31 revealed a tumor marker of a high 145.7, I was able to remain calm and factor in what my doctors had told me about the role stress might play and to take into account my recent furlough from supplements during the two-week hospital stay.

The therapist taught me how to use visual imagery; to block out ambient distractions and focus on a specific problem; to use deep breathing exercises; to do an exercise wherein only one part of the body is relaxed at a time; and perhaps most important, how to employ self-hypnosis.

To be sure, it wasn't a quick fix as my stomach upsets continued and I still had the muscle spasm of the rib cage that had started a few weeks ago in the hospital. Furthermore, on November 12, my husband's birthday, I found myself back in the hospital, this time for five days suffering from another blood clot of the left leg that had broken loose into three parts and lodged in my lungs. My doctor and the nurses told me that this was a "close one" as such a clot dispersal was often fatal. And here I learned that I would be on blood thinner the rest of my life. Still, I felt that without this hypnotherapy I would be having a more difficult time dealing with all this.

My weight loss continued even while in the hospital and one day following my release it dropped to just over 113 pounds, the lowest since contracting cancer; in fact, the lowest since my early teen years. My appearance was so deathly, that even my hypnotherapist seemed disquieted by it and in my next session had taken an even more focused tack. Despite the intensity of the session, I felt unhurried and even more deeply relaxed.

After having me seat myself in a very comfortable leather recliner, the therapist had me close my eyes and place my hands on my "tummy" and in a very soft and soothing tone had me go through deeper and deeper stages of relaxation. While counting backwards from 10 to zero very slowly, suggestions were made that I was becoming more and more in touch with the "mind of my body" and that its various organs were also becoming more relaxed by "letting go" of any tension. He slowly detailed specific organs and other parts especially those involved with digestion but included as well the musculature of my rib cage to reduce its spasms, and my throat to reduce the soreness that had lingered from the NG tube used with the hospital stomach pump weeks earlier.

And at the end of the session I was feeling very calm and experienced a return of my appetite! When I mentioned this to the therapist he smiled broadly and suggested that going out and having lunch might be appropriate. John and I went to Red Lobster and for once I ordered more than just a baked potato. It was a full meal, thank you, and even though I couldn't quite finish it, I couldn't have been happier. Although the soreness remained in my rib area and throat, these parts also seemed to celebrate, the pain having subsided just enough to allow some feeling of comfort.

On December 5, 1995, John and I had two important errands to perform: one was to go in for my CA-125 blood draw, the results of which would form the tumor marker and be ready in about a week; the second was to attend as guests a class at the University or Arizona Medical School normally taught by Andrew Weil, a well-known M.D. who included alternative medicine in his practice and instruction. My hypnotherapist had been called on to take over the class in Dr. Weil's absence and had planned on using my medical experiences in explaining and demonstrating hypnotherapy.

This was the first time John and I had set foot in a medical school classroom and it wasn't what we had expected. The amphitheater-styled room seemed quite small and had a rather untidy appearance as the chairs were arranged haphazardly. In a word, the physical setting looked so ordinary and with some of the medical students coming in and opening their lunch bags, the room appeared all the more utilitarian. Of course, this class met at noon and it was the last day of the semester. And perhaps most significant, their regular instructor was absent and this may also explain why students wandered in and out from time to time.

But the students became very attentive and remained in their seats when shark cartilage was mentioned, but the instructional plans went out the window. My therapist opened the class and explained his professional function and introduced me as someone who was undergoing hypnotherapy. He had asked me to talk some about my medical history and why I had sought his therapeutic help. By this time in 1995, my story had become a long one but I did try to keep it as short as possible. However, when I mentioned the role of shark cartilage in my cancer treatment protocol, the students straightened up and zeroed in on this therapy raising question after question. Any hopes of getting back on track were abandoned and the rest of the period was devoted to discussing the possible merits of this weird-sounding cartilage treatment.

What became abundantly clear was the striking differences among these medical students in both their personalities and outlook. Most of them asked probing questions concerning why I was so sure it was the shark cartilage that had produced the beneficial results I had only briefly sketched and most seemed very impressed that my long-standing rheumatoid arthritis had vanished along with the cancer pain and that my CA-125 tumor marker also responded favorably. But when I elaborated on why I had gone off the shark cartilage for some eight months of repeated surgeries and, consequently, that my tumor marker was now on the rise, some very sharp differences of opinion erupted.

Stepping in late was a small group of older students, some appearing to be practicing physicians. They remained in the back of the room and especially scowled when I touched upon the role of cartilage antiangiogenesis in making our decision not to chance having it interfere with my surgical healing. One suggested that I had simply bought into something that offered hope and had the magic powder been made up of finely ground sand, my responses to it would have been the same.

My husband, John, pointed out that I had high hopes for my

three courses of chemotherapy and they still failed; that the benefits of the cartilage were surprising because I actually had little hope that this approach would work; and that my apparently metastatic and terminal brain tumor turned out encapsulated and benign – all facts heavily weighing against a placebo effect. But one young woman seated up front smiled radiantly and suggested that since my arthritis symptoms disappeared so early, we probably did come to have more faith in the cartilage from that point on. Of course, this was true but the class ended before John had a chance to explain that we knew this initial benefit didn't guarantee later success against cancer. But to our surprise, a large portion of the class spilled out into the hallway after us and we did have a chance to talk more. These students who were mostly quite young had shown considerable openness and enthusiasm for my novel treatment. My therapist also seemed exceedingly pleased with the way things had turned out.

But only two more hypnotherapy sessions were to follow and just months later we learned that this man's wife had died. And it was especially sad because I knew he had done his very best for her.

* * * *

On December 7, 1995, just two days following the visit to Dr. Weil's class, we were looking forward to watching an afternoon talk show on Fox Television. About a month earlier, I had received a phone call from a volunteer connected to Dr. I. William Lane's organization asking if I would be willing, if chosen, to appear on the "Gabrielle Show." My answer was yes, but only days later John had to call and tell them I had to return to the hospital (on November 12 to dissolve blood clot segments in my leg and lungs) and that it would be impossible to travel to California for the program's taping. Of course, this was another disappointment but one of the producers of the show called and informed John that this December 7 program was the one I had missed being on and so we were eager to see it.

Because there was so much gratuitous clapping and noise-making encouraged by the host for any good news divulged, especially by the invited cancer survivors, our impression of the show was not all that positive. However, John had taped the program and when we watched it again it became apparent that the show's producers were probably operating within the constraints imposed by a popular culture that tends to value entertainment over substance, and even senseless controversy over reasoned analysis. Thus, the show viewed while mindful of this context actually seemed quite balanced. And again, John and I were reminded not to allow superficial influences to close off sources of information. In fact, one guest pointed out that cancer information gleaned many years before on another talk show had saved her son's life.

While the show made an effort to include many of the unconventional approaches to cancer treatment, two seemed to stand out. As we had expected, one of them was the use of shark cartilage. The other was the use of antineoplastons, naturally occurring protein-like substance that had been discovered about 30 years ago by a prominent and now Houston-based physician and researcher, Stanislaw Burzynski, M.D., Ph.D. Perhaps this distinguished Polish-born doctor could be faulted for not bringing other nontoxic therapeutic agents into play along side of the antineoplastons in treating his large body of mostly terminal patients. Nevertheless, his treatment protocols have been shown to work in many of these "hopeless" cases to the extent that the Food and Drug Administration has lately been overseeing the protocols, though very begrudgingly.

Despite general recognition that this therapy is sometimes effective, the producers of the "Gabrielle Show" could not find one doctor (apparently from among M.D.s) who was willing to appear on the show with Dr. Burzynski. In fact, one of the 25 doctors contacted said of him, "He is an antichrist, he is an Adolf Hitler." Even though this audience may have been somewhat jaded, it moaned upon hearing this particular defamation of Dr. Burzynski. Interestingly, Burzynski's father had been jailed by the Nazis in Poland and the doctor himself had refused early on to join the then-dominant Communist Party of Poland despite great pressure to do so.

And now in these free United States, bureaucrats and government prosecutors were trying to imprison this Texas doctor perhaps for life principally because some of his patients had crossed state lines in taking home their medicine!!! And the patients themselves (along with the good doctor) had to take to the streets and to the courts to fight off their own government in a 15-year struggle so that they might live.

If you the reader thought the Tuskegee syphilis experiment which left poor blacks untreated was medieval or thought the callous treatment of Gulf War veterans apparently impaired by errant chemical clouds was unconscionable, wait until you learn the full details of the Burzynski case. You will come to fully understand why one poll in *USA Today* (Pew Research Center), suggested that only six percent of the population had "a lot" of trust in government. (Of course, Burzynski's patients largely realize it is big pharmaceutical money influencing big government that is behind much of their grief. *The Burzynski Breakthrough* by Thomas D. Elias is one book that chronicles in chilling and riveting detail the full Burzynski story.)

* * * *

The "Gabrielle Show" had brought on Dr. I. William Lane along with a nun who had successfully treated her malignancy with shark cartilage and all things considered we felt that the program had made a positive contribution toward a better understanding of natural, nontoxic cancer therapies. But my own battle against cancer had become even less certain as the most recent blood draw of December 5 revealed a higher tumor marker. My CA-125 had risen from 145.7 to 188.5 and John and I still wonder why we hadn't become more alarmed by this now obvious trend. Most probably we were still basking in the glow of so much good news rendered by the surgeons who had found no cancer.

In telling us of the tumor marker's rise, the nurse's expression was neutral and she said little except to suggest that because of all that had happened to me, its meaning was still not that clear. John who tends to analyze everything, actually charted the marker's upward progression and having established curvilinearity, concluded that my tumor marker might well have been in the upper 80's when my abdominal organs were freed October 4 and the two surgeons still could find no cancer. It seemed as though everyone around me, including John, was mystified, but I knew what was happening, and yet I didn't assert myself.

Then came December 14 and I experienced morning diarrhea. At first I didn't think much of it but it soon made intermittent returns only to become chronic. Although I was absorbed in Christmas preparations, I still sensed that things were coming to a head and right after the holidays, January 2, 1996, John and I rushed to the lab for another blood draw. And a week later tension filled the cancer clinic as we were told that my marker had risen to 236.2 thus indicating along with the diarrhea that the cancer was back. Now the oncology nurse who had always impressed us as being very knowledgeable spoke bluntly, saying, "Ovarian cancer is very good at hiding." Obviously my intuition was right, and when John told the nurse that I was going to begin taking the shark cartilage again, I couldn't wait to get started.

* * * *

Because the internist seemed more favorably disposed toward my taking the bovine cartilage compared to the shark variety, we were perhaps swayed to view its potential more favorably than it deserved. But impressions die hard and John had called the well-known cancer author and researcher, Ralph W. Moss, Ph.D., to ask among other things if he had ever known someone to successfully combine the therapies. And he had. So John felt that combining the two forms of cartilage at least for a time would do no harm. Besides writing such books as *The Cancer Industry*, and *Cancer Therapy*, Dr. Moss also supervised an inexpensive information service based on his research and we had subscribed to it.

Upon receiving my latest tumor marker, the highest ever, my oncologist, of course, was concerned and on January 17, John and I were in his office. An intern brought in my voluminous records and was quick to suggest that alternative therapies seldom work. Although he was soft spoken and rather bland in manner, he quietly dominated the session and cited several cases he knew of which supported his conclusion. And when my oncologist stepped in, the general tenor of the exchanges continued as my doctor said little. We discerned that my oncologist had expected more of the bovine cartilage as had my internist and was similarly disappointed. And when John said that my surgical healing was well along and we thus felt it safe to start taking the shark cartilage again, my oncologist nodded approvingly. Surprisingly, even the quietly outspoken intern seemed to agree that I could not withstand more treatments of the toxic kind.

Sometimes I think John and I take turns assuming the role of worrywart and now it was his turn. Even though I was slowly gaining weight and generally feeling better, my diarrhea continued without let up and poor John concentrated on the negative and was unable to see the forest beyond the trees. And he started to pester me to do more. But what?

John was more worried than sure, but he had noted that Dr. Ralph Moss in the research report recently mailed to us was impressed with a variation of the Kelley program. The original program advanced by William D. Kelley, D.D.S. emphasized the use of pancreatic enzymes along with sound nutrition and detoxification.

Dr. Kelley who was a dentist by training had developed this program well over a quarter-century ago in an effort to repulse his own pancreatic cancer and because this nontoxic approach did appear to succeed, it was viciously suppressed. Now, John thought it would do no harm to incorporate it in my health program. Another less intensive variation of the Kelley therapy had already been instituted by my naturopathic doctor at the same time I had originally started on the shark cartilage, but John convinced me in consultation with the doctor to seek out a nutritionist who specialized in this approach. The nutritionist had ordered a blood test and urinalysis for me and accordingly my health program was further refined just a couple of weeks before my next CA-125 tumor marker assay.

chapter twelve

Back on Track

The first months of 1996 found me feeling better and eating more. My weight had climbed steadily and was now above 120 pounds. And at the end of February, refinements in my supplement protocol favoring among other changes a broader range of digestive enzymes seemed to soothe my digestion, at least somewhat. But adding shark cartilage to the mix was a bit of a challenge.

As you might remember, we (actually, John) decided I should also continue on the bovine capsules, at least for a while. This ambitious regimen saw me taking seven doses of cartilage spread throughout the day and two of them (shark) were by retention enemas and quite time consuming. The five oral doses required an empty stomach and the logistics for this was problematic since I also needed quite a number of smaller meals daily.

It was 10 PM Tuesday January 9, 1996, when I again started taking the shark cartilage and although we ran out of the BeneFin powder for a day or so along the way, I averaged an intake of 64.65 grams per day for the eight weeks ending Thursday, March 7, the date of my next CA-125 blood draw.

We had every intention of maintaining a higher dosage level of the shark cartilage, but considering my weight of about 125 pounds, I was taking the minimum amount often recommended for the control of cancer.

Since it took my HMO's lab close to a week to assay my blood sample and send out the result, we did not know whether it would be available on Tuesday five days after the blood draw when we returned to Tucson for my GYN cancer support meeting. My group met at the cancer clinic and often John would go upstairs to my oncologist's office and ask the nurse for the tumor marker. But this time John was panicky and insisted that I go up with him though I could be late for the support meeting. The nurse was just behind the reception counter and recognized us immediately as we stepped forward. When we asked her for my tumor marker, she nodded, "You're in luck... they just came in." The nurse disappeared for a minute and then glided out toward us rather triumphantly and sporting a distinct air of satisfaction showed John and me the CA-125 number as written on my records. It was 95.6 and John sighed noisily.

The nurse stood looking at us in sheer wonderment. My first comment centered on how the shark cartilage was the only treatment that had worked for me. But John was concerned that the lab may have made a mistake. "Not likely," said the nurse. "When there is an unexpected change like this, the lab double checks it." And then she explained that this drop from 236.2 in just over nine weeks was highly dramatic.

John remarked that I had returned to the BeneFin powder during the last eight weeks between blood draws and extrapolatory calculations might reveal the tumor marker decline actually began from a higher level of about 250. I am not sure that the nurse absorbed John's rather crazy sounding analysis as she obviously had questions.

"What did you have along with the shark cartilage powder?" she asked. And when I started to rattle off the long list of other natural substances that I had long been taking, she had me halt. No, she was only interested in knowing whether I had also been on radiation, chemotherapy, or even hormonal therapy. When I told her I had never been on radiation and had been off of chemotherapy since June of 1994 and hormonal therapies since April of 1995, she nodded positively and said something that both John and I failed to fathom at the time. "Don't ever let someone talk you out of taking this nontoxic cartilage powder or anything else you find helpful," was the nurse's stern warning. "Don't let someone do it, even if there are impressive letters after the person's name."

As she departed the waiting room and closed the door behind her, we both walked away with the warm feeling that she was truly trying to help us. And our puzzlement over her stern warning would be cleared up in the months ahead.

* * * *

To say we savored this salubrious marker represents quite an understatement especially for John who now revealed, "I think you're going to make it." And not even my morning diarrhea which remained a daily annoyance significantly tempered his revived outlook. Not that he threw caution to the wind, either.

John being John, only grudgingly had he agreed to my forgoing the Essiac tea briefly mentioned earlier and which intermittently had been a part of my daily routine almost from the beginning of my renewed cancer struggle that started in mid 1994.

Originally an Ojibwa (Chippewa) Indian brew made from herbs found in the North American rainforest belt, John and I had spent considerable time mixing these same ingredients and brewing them on our kitchen range. This Essiac brew was interchanged with a similar blend that my naturopathic physician labeled, "A Hoxsey-like Formula." Even though this latter blend was already made up, I also had difficulty retaining it as part my regimen because of everything else I was taking. When I suggested to John that the bovine cartilage might be expendable as well, he cautioned that forgoing one medicament at a time would provide at least some indication of what helped me and what didn't. And as far as we could tell, the elimination of these two similar and alternated treatments made little or no apparent difference. But still, they could have provided an underlying enhancement of my immune system.

Although I had just contracted the flu, in mid March we

nevertheless telephoned a Portland, Oregon naturopathic physician and cartilage researcher by the name of Martin Milner. We had read a research article of his and thought he might well be an exceptional source of information. After reviewing my medical history and cartilage protocol with him, he suggested that I be sure to take the shark cartilage on an empty stomach usually an hour before meals and, interestingly, to increase the dosage. He seemed amused by our great interest in alternative medicine noting that when people discover that nontoxic approaches can work, they become all the more receptive to the field in general. All in all, I found his friendly reassurance comforting and we were destined to meet him in about six months.

It is interesting to note that my being highly receptive to various avenues of support no doubt makes it easier for me to deal with the cancer compared to John who tends to face the adversity in a brooding and more solitary way. This is not to suggest, however, that I was having an easy time of it.

The gastrointestinal upsets were still with me and about this time I began having slight headaches every three or four days. Naturally, this was worrisome especially in light of just a year ago having the brain tumor removed.

During this period I had attended eight weekly "holistic" sessions which dealt with the stress often associated with cancer. The program included breathing exercises; stretching the body in various ways; yoga; meditation; and other even more exotic approaches to stress management. It is difficult to establish cause-and-effect relationships, of course, but after three weeks my headaches vanished and I know of doctors who would likely suggest that my willingness to participate in such a program and continue doing the exercises at home might have indeed played a positive role in this and some of the other outcomes I've enjoyed. Although John seemed willing to read and wait for me outside, he showed little interest in the program otherwise, and because of the great number of women who participated, the very few men who chose to mingle actually stood out.

Of course, all of those in my GYN cancer support group were women and I believe just about every member experienced some form of relief through the unique reciprocity of understanding that existed, an empathy that could not be matched in any other social setting. And I could tell that many in the group were showing a keen but often cautious interest in my case. And a TV news magazine segment perfectly illustrated why caution of a special kind is so necessary, especially for those suffering a life threatening illness.

* * * *

Needless to say, by this time we were taking more than a casual interest in health matters, particularly those related to cancer, and our television viewing habits had been influenced considerably. On March 22, 1996, there was one TV report which struck especially John as singularly poignant in disclosing the quagmire desperately ill people frequently had to slog through, often with little hope of extrication.

The ABC News magazine, "20/20" told the story of a young boy who suffered from pediatric epilepsy and often had innumerable seizures daily. The conventional treatments the boy received seemed to do as much harm as the seizures themselves. Despite the very best conventional medical advice this country had to offer, the parents were finally faced with having their boy undergo especially desperate – and dangerous – surgery. And strangely, their own desperation drove them to the library.

It was here in the quiet ranks of books and journals that the parents discovered a remedy developed in the roaring 1920's but silently received by the medical community because it only involved a complex dietary change and it hadn't been formally tested by the pharmaceutical industry! But the clinical evidence showed that this Ketogenic Diet (which, surprisingly, is high in fat) stopped the seizures in about one-third of epileptic children and significantly helped the conditions of another third. Overall, these outcomes are far better than those results obtained by conventional drugs and surgeries and are far less expensive.

Fortunately, the parents discounted the diet's medical detractors and took their boy to the John Hopkins Medical Center and Hospital, one of the few places using this alternative remedy. And the outcome was spectacular: upwards of 90 seizures a day were reduced to zero!

Unbelievably, this unconventional treatment had languished in obscurity for almost 70 years and may continue to do so. But to the credit of the ABC Network, less than a year later in 1997 the story was told in a full-length docudrama entitled, "... First Do No Harm," starring Meryl Streep as the mother. It should be remembered that most media organizations must depend on their advertisers to maintain the bottom line and to be sure big advertisers do often influence program content. Therefore, it is amazing that this story aired in such a big way or even at all.

* * * *

John and I had learned through our own experience that it is not that easy to discount the recommendations of medical figures and go your own way as did these parents. We had an idea of the uncertainty they felt and of the questions they must have asked themselves, most no doubt revolving around whether theirs was the best option. Then, too, these parents must have experienced profound relief and even surprise when the option chosen actually worked and continued to do so. Taking responsibility for your own health or for that of a loved one involves facing such a forbidding and lonely road that few are actually able to take it. And even at this point in my own recovery, we had to face this reality and be content to let seriously ill acquaintances and friends with cancer make their own decisions even if they choose to simply wait for death. One must realize that this is what most of us have been conditioned to do: see your medical doctor and do as he says, regardless. And, indeed, that is what many of us end up doing.

We had also belatedly chosen an unconventional path stemming from our own desperation and this path could have odds for success similar to those of the Ketogenic Diet. And now my diarrhea had ceased in mid-April and my favorable CA-125 tumor marker of April 31, which dropped from 95.6 to 70.5, gave ample evidence that my shark cartilage therapy was continuing its beneficial work. While my husband and I were elated, it was tempered some by yet more problems.

* * * *

During these early months of 1996, I continued to have monthly blood draws to uncover my "protime" (the time it takes for my blood to coagulate to stop bleeding). It might be remembered that I had been put on the blood thinner coumadin "for life" in order to help preclude blood clots from recurring in my chemo-damaged left leg. An unwelcome side effect of the medication is bruising, and black-and-blue marks would mysteriously pop up especially on my arms and legs and often last for ages. As well, precautions against excessive bleeding had to be taken for medical procedures including most dental work.

As my luck would have it, on May 23 a lower crown broke loose and the supporting molar had all but disintegrated. My dentist was openly disturbed by this structural weakness and said it could have been caused by past chemotherapy. He examined all my teeth exhaustively but felt the need to send me to two specialists for further examination as perhaps my other teeth were similarly weakened. But even if this didn't prove true, the now defunct molar still presented a remedial problem. As matters worked out, my remaining teeth seemed solid enough so that the very time consuming installation of a dental implant to replace my molar seemed to be the best option despite its expense. Unbelievably, at about the same time a mysterious pain developed.

The day following my molar breakup, a severe pain worked

its way across the bridge of my nose to envelop the areas around both eyes and ultimately to skip down and affect the very bottom of my chin. The pain was accompanied by considerable swelling especially across the bridge of my nose.

My dentist said that the lower right collapsed molar (which had yet to be pulled out) had nothing to do with the pain which was centered on the left side of my nose. The pain and swelling was so unrelenting, though, that I wound up in urgent care. The doctor there was also mystified as he could find no infection or other apparent cause even after a very exhaustive examination. He prescribed an antibiotic just in case an infection was somehow missed and sent John and me on our way. And in about a week the pain and swelling completely disappeared but, of course, the mystery remained.

* * * *

There was no concealing my weight, however, as it had been rising rapidly and was now above 140 pounds. My internist had viewed any weight increase as potentially beneficial but unhappily an abdominal distention was now magnified. The routine removal of portions of the omentum support tissue during my hysterectomy plus the effects of subsequent abdominal surgeries (and, no doubt, advancing age) had produced this now more prominent bloating. But this deformity did little to moderate our deep satisfaction from my July 1 tumor marker which declined from 70.5 to only 46.1, now much closer to the normal range of 35 and below. But it took only a few days for a not-so-old worry to make its comeback.

The pain and swelling across the bridge of my nose returned in much the same manner it came in the previous occurrence except that the pain's locus was now on the right side and didn't involve any portion of my chin. I managed to see my internist about this episode and he too seemed baffled. Radiographs were negative and my doctor prescribed the antibiotic used to treat the previous occurrence. The pain's center migrated to the opposite side of my nose and then the pain vanished entirely.

Again, it must be emphasized that the acute awareness of one's cancer very seldom vacations but unceasingly works to undermine one's confidence in whatever good news that comes along. Looking back on these mysterious episodes is essentially untroubling; however, the same could not be said of them while they were actually happening even though we knew they were not necessarily serious.

On July 17, John and I were back to see the oncologist for my semiannual examination and he certainly didn't seem to see dark clouds in the unexplained episodes I had suffered. In fact, he looked down at the numbers and spoke very softly, as though to himself, "236.2... 95.6... 70.5... 46.1... can only be explained by..." Slowly moving his head to and fro in deep concentration, he abruptly turned to the both of us and emphasized, "Something like this just doesn't happen out of the blue." Apparently bound by time constraints, he quickened the pace but again asked John about where he obtained the cartilage, its cost, and its dosage requirements. Following this brief exchange, he arose and asked John to do him a favor by detailing my cartilage treatment protocol in writing and giving the particulars to his nurse (which John did a week later).

* * * *

On the whole, I had been feeling better which is not to say I was back to normal or anywhere near it. It was just that not too long ago I had gotten used to being almost continually ill and now being sick half of the time was quite a relief. But some violent gastrointestinal upsets returned for a brief period and reminded me that the more severe effects of the chemotherapy I had had were not going to bow out all that graciously.

Meanwhile, because of the declining tumor markers, I began reducing the shark cartilage intake despite my weight gains advising the opposite. In the weeks before my latest marker of 46.1, I averaged 72.7 grams of the shark cartilage daily; during the weeks following, the average daily dosage was down to 59.6 grams. The dental implant work done in this latter period was only a minor consideration. Simply, I just wasn't listening to John. But John wasn't as concerned about the reduction as he would have been had I not been taking the recommended dosage of the bovine cartilage. Even though my instincts told me the bovine capsules weren't helping, John's stubborn nature still prevailed, at least for now.

Another of John's habits, that of writing letters to the editor, came into play about this time as a rather lengthy report of his concerning my case was printed in the 1996 August/September issue of the *Townsend Letter*, a journal purporting to be "The Examiner of Medical Alternatives." In it John had suggested that if it hadn't been for Dr. I. William Lane's persistence and penchant for publicity, I wouldn't be alive today and that no one ever has the right to keep a potentially lifesaving, nontoxic treatment hidden behind a sealed agreement (which is sometimes done to enhance profits or one's status with the pharmaceutical cartel).

But the unsealing of my August 20 blood draw results showed a CA-125 tumor marker up almost five points from my very auspicious marker of seven weeks ago. It was now up to 49.9 and its portent hardly worried us. For one thing, I had failed to eliminate the digestive and pancreatic enzymes from my diet for the three days prior to the blood draw as had been instructed by my nutrition specialist. And we also knew that other factors could throw the marker off and so the happier prospects of again attending the Pasadena, California Convention of the Cancer Control Society, this time over the 1996 Labor Day weekend, absorbed so much more of our attention.

chapter thirteen

Perseverance

It is hard to admit that John and I had debated, though very briefly, whether the potential benefits of attending the 1996 Cancer Control Society Convention was worth our making the necessary 550-mile trip to Pasadena, California. But surprisingly, although this traditional Labor Day weekend repeat featured many of the same speakers heard last year, the setting still seemed remarkably fresh to us. In fact, some of the repetition proved helpful because of the many revelations we missed our first time around. Perhaps most remarkably, many of the repeat speakers being on the leading edge of clinical and sometimes formal research themselves seemed to have used the interim to grow professionally. In this following year, however, we did sense some negatives not especially noted before.

For one, a follow-the-leader tendency seemed to prevail perhaps based more on individual prestige differences than necessity. The newest wrinkle in alternative medicine similarly had to be at least mentioned by just about every speaker even to the point of straying from the subject at hand. Last year (1995) it was shark cartilage, this next year it was bovine cartilage advanced by "the father of cartilage therapy," John F. Prudden, M.D. And seemingly there was some contentiousness as a number of speakers suggested that the bovine cartilage might be a stronger anti-tumor agent than the shark variety. (But for me, this assertion seemed pointless as both could be used together and one might work for some people and not others). But the argument seemed to be settled by members of the audience.

Although the audience was made up largely of professionals

in the health care field, the general public was also invited and probably comprised half of the attendees. And on Sunday, mid-day, a speaker who was to cover "The Successful Use of Bovine Cartilage in Cancer, Arthritis and Autoimmune Diseases" did not answer the call and the subject was dropped without an apparent sound from the audience.

The next midday, I. William Lane, Ph.D., was scheduled to speak of "The Latest Research and Clinical Trials on Shark Cartilage" and when it was announced he was unavailable, loud moans coursed through the audience somewhat unsettling the emcee who had to yell, "Wait!" to restore calm. Another shark cartilage researcher was to make the presentation and it was Dr. Martin Milner the Oregon naturopathic physician whom we had consulted by telephone some six months earlier.

The somewhat diminutive doctor sported an expression warmly reminiscent of an agile cat that had just finished his favorite course for dinner. He immediately got down to business, his carrousel projector flashing image after image charting the results of clinical trials and showing the stark remains of cartilage-treated tumors. In answering closing questions he knocked down suggestions that the human body is unable to absorb shark cartilage and then quickly left the podium as he had a plane to catch. But the crowd of about 30 people who trailed behind surrounded him in the inner hotel foyer and now he appeared more like the mouse who saw no way out.

One young woman wanted to thank him because the cartilage spared her the need of a colostomy to try and slow her "terminal" colon cancer. And when she said that she could only afford 30 grams of the shark cartilage per day but it still stabilized her cancer, the doctor looked at his watch but decided to stay. Visibly troubled, he warned his rapt listeners that this propitious result on such a low dosage was rare and almost always only a larger dosage schedule brought success. The very few people who benefit from a low dosage level, he explained, are usually very sensitive to many other substances, including aspirin.

While quite a number here just wanted to report their success in using the therapy, perhaps a greater number had terminal cancer or had a loved one who was desperate. One was a small elderly woman whose palsied hands made her note taking slow and uncertain. The doctor directed her to a point directly in front of him and extended his arms protectively from time to time to guard her from the normal movements of the much larger people around her. Apparently, her equally aged husband had terminal prostate cancer and the doctor made sure she managed to take down the particulars needed to initiate therapy. He warned her that the husband had to be willing to do it as she couldn't take the cartilage for him.

Despite all this desperation clouding the area, a woman behind a nearby booth selling something, frowned and complained that the group was blocking the way for any potential customers who might happen by (something unlikely while the main conference was in session). And this person was of an age whereby she could have been the daughter of this desperate old woman. Indeed, even in this small way, the dollar and its attendant self-interest is shown to be alive and well! Historically, this is to be expected.

* * * *

It needs to be emphasized that of the various economic and political systems vying for our allegiance on the world stage, democracy and the free enterprise system have triumphed. Central planning in the political realm may appear nicely focused and organized, but it fails to take full advantage of individual initiative and thereby results in stagnation and ultimately, disintegration. The same holds true of monopolies and cartels, central planning mechanisms created primarily to satisfy economic interests. But the more successful open systems which have served our country so well seem inherently messy and thus often invite both necessary and unnecessary controls. The broadly encompassing alternative arena because it is based more on the free enterprise model, is not nearly as reassuring to most health seekers because to venture into it requires one to be a very careful consumer. And, sadly, most of us would rather hand over that awesome responsibility to someone else, regardless of the consequences.

Thus, our venture into this realm certainly was not always consoling but as with many people here at this cancer convention, we became advocates of the "Access to Medical Treatment Act," the explanation of which was now and had been a central part of convention programs.

True, what was not enumerated in favor of health freedom at the Constitutional Convention in Philadelphia way back in 1787 hadn't made that much difference during our country's earlier history because no one economic health interest had gained the ascendancy. But by the early 1900s, matters had changed so much that today we are saddled with the sight of terminal cancer patients having to travel to foreign countries to seek out needed non-pharmaceutical treatments while we attempt to convince those outside our borders that we are free and thus worthy of emulation.

However, as a people we do have a right to assemble and to petition our representatives in government as well as have considerable freedom of expression which, sadly, is severely restricted in the health area – again, another legacy of the cartel's big money.

So now, John, and especially I as a recovered "terminal" cancer patient, have been called upon to write and telephone and fax and e-mail local, state and national politicians to encourage them to simply legislate medical freedom. And we recovered patients as well as the others gathered here at this 1996 Cancer Control Society Convention should not be the only ones who contemplate our Statue of Liberty and other symbols of liberty and ask how could such a precious freedom be stripped from the American landscape so easily. Perhaps Edmund Burke gave the answer when he said: "The only thing necessary for the triumph of evil is for good men to do nothing."

* * * *

On our way home from the convention, we discussed the proceedings extensively. The well-known author, Julian Whitaker, M.D., spoke this year and since he had been an outspoken supporter of the beleaguered Dr. Stanislaw Burzynski, we were surprised he hadn't also brought on the government's wrath. In fact, several of Burzynski's loyal patients gave a short presentation – as did I, a few hours later.

John had decided last year that I would speak during the "The Recovered Patients' Presentation" which was a popular feature. My dear husband administered an adroit shove and I was first in line to tell my two-minutes worth. "Well, everyone including the media paid full attention to you," John said. Of course he said this and with a smile hinting such an outcome was unexpected. Regardless, a number of people did tell me my short talk was informative.

The 20 or so recovered patients who spoke represented a variety of nontoxic therapies. Many had gone through programs involving a number of natural treatments simultaneously administered. And most had been labeled "terminal" by their conventional doctors.

But for John and me, the highlight of the conference was an announcement by Dr. Milner that a Japanese clinical trial using shark cartilage and other natural immunotherapies had produced an initial 70 percent remission in otherwise terminal cancer patients. This news helped me face the problems that still lurked before me at home.

* * * *

On balance, attending the conference was a delight but I still had pains and upsets there. Even the old hoarseness stemming from the hospital NG tube inserted months earlier had made a return. But now at home the eerie pain that had plagued me earlier was back. And this time it wasn't the bridge of my nose involved, but my thumb! Again, it was unlike my old arthritic torment and was especially severe with any exertion or pressure. However, after about three weeks – puff – it disappeared.

Meanwhile, my implant dentistry was continuing and I did cease taking the shark cartilage for a few days before and after any serious dental work. But my general health was improving perhaps aided by my nutritional efforts and by September 19 my weight was up to a rather hefty 147 pounds! It took some doing, but I convinced John that my ingesting the bovine cartilage was superfluous and after October 7, I ceased taking it.

About this time, a woman with a warm, sympathetic voice telephoned John about the *Townsend Letter* report he had written and she had noted the unusual twists and turns my case had taken. And this woman, Marian Murphy, had used shark cartilage and like me had vanquished a mortal brain tumor. Only a part of her large tumor could be surgically excised and she had been left with little hope. But a nutritionist pointed Marian toward the cartilage therapy and in time her tumor shrank and became inactive. Her case was featured in a 1996 video documentary produced by Cartilage Consultants, Inc., entitled; "Shark Cartilage: A Promise Kept."

Happy to be alive, she at first informally talked to others with similar experiences and then was employed by Cartilage Consultants, Inc., of New Jersey to develop an international information and support system for cancer victims who were either taking clinical grade shark cartilage or contemplating doing so. And after inquiring about my medical history and related records, she asked if my name might be included in the telephone network so that others could benefit from my cancer experiences.

Having already joined groups who help cancer victims in need of information and encouragement, my answer was an immediate yes. And considering the providential favor I had experienced, I don't know how I could have said no to this or any other volunteer effort. In many ways my life had been enriched by the scores of cancer patients I had already talked to.

* * * *

Months earlier (May 19, 1996), I showed my husband a very brief article from Knight-Ridder reports tucked away in an obscure part of the newspaper. John Hopkins University researchers reported that a substance in shark livers, squalamine, markedly slows the formation of blood vessels that nourish solid brain tumors. And the researchers concluded that this antiangiogenic action may help fight these malignancies.

John's great interest in this report was now apparent as he sweet-talked me into adding a new product, ImmunoFin (Lane Labs, NJ, distributor), to my daily regimen. Consequently, six capsules containing "a proprietary all natural concentrate of shark liver oil" were added daily starting October 20. I had argued against this addition, but two days later when my CA-125 tumor marker had jumped from 49.9 to 72.9 and within only five weeks, heftier dosages of the shark cartilage quickly became a reality. In fact, I ended up with six or seven doses daily and again I was taking one in the middle of the night!

We had gone through these "bounces" before but I couldn't get John to calm down and listen to reason. I knew the cartilage was working but pinpointing exactly how I knew was a problem. And John wasn't about to buy any "nonsense" about my intuition. God only knows what else I might be taking should the marker rise again and needless to say I was getting worried not only because of John's behavior but because two and sometimes three of the daily doses were taken by retention enema and I knew there had to be a limit.

In the weeks before this troublesome 72.9 marker, I had only averaged an intake of about 55 grams of cartilage per day because of extensive dental work. Soon after this high marker, my average daily intake of BeneFin powder was pumped up drastically averaging about 104 grams daily. At nearly 150 pounds, my minimum cartilage intake should have been nearer 75 grams daily. Therefore, the prior period was deficient.

I had completely forgotten about the dental work and being off of the cartilage for a week, but my medical diary came to the rescue. (Surprisingly, though, one contrarious researcher later observed any dental or other type of surgery could actually undergo improved recovery through the ingestion of shark cartilage!)

As previously mentioned, some people have had to take as high as one gram of cartilage powder per pound of body weight and that level would require my ingesting nearly 150 grams per day!

But to my relief, such a high level proved unnecessary. The CA-125 of December 3 was down smartly, thank you, and I savored the tumor marker of 37.2 (down from 72.9) as though it were sweeter than candy. But John soured my joy somewhat by insisting I continue taking the 104 grams of cartilage daily. (But just between you and me, John can be quite excitable and I quietly lowered the dosage to about 93 grams daily and managed to get away with it. The power of positive thinking!)

* * * *

The power of negativism, on the other hand, was alive and functioning. Even the terminal patients who were telephoning me had often waited until it was too late to really do anything because of negative influences. One woman I heard from had to administer the cartilage and similar substances to her cancer stricken mother very discretely because of opposition from her father. And some medical doctors were openly hostile. They were more likely to confront John than me and a typical conversation went something like this:

Doctor: I had two patients who took that cartilage stuff and they died anyway.

John: What brand were they using and how much were they taking daily?

Doctor: I have no idea.

John: Your two patients were no doubt terminal, how long did they have to live when they started taking it?

Doctor: A month or two.

John: Many people start too late, take too little and use a brand which isn't processed for cancer control.

Doctor: It wouldn't matter. The stuff doesn't work anyway.

A listener might be troubled by such a lack of insight yet forget that many "good" doctors simply have the ability to deftly jump through hoops and parrot information. While such traits may serve these high professionals well in both school and consensus medicine, they preclude reasoned judgments especially when perceived self-interest is added to the mix. A woman's cartilage-controlled pancreatic cancer favorably discussed on a TV talk show, prompted one doctor to caution terminal cancer patients not to chance going outside of conventional medicine! Now the stern warning given months ago by the oncology nurse against responding to impressive sounding "authorities" came to be fully understood – and appreciated!

* * * *

December of 1996, is hardly a month to be remembered, at least not the same way as December, 1995, and happily so. But the new month did feature some pain. It was my thumb again and this time the affliction favored one swollen and worn out vein often used for the infusion of past therapeutic poisons. Perhaps because I soaked the thumb frequently in warm water and Epsom salts, it responded nicely and within a week the pain vanished. The favorable tumor marker at the beginning of the month as already mentioned had put me in a more positive frame of mind and I was ready to face the 1996 holiday season now just ahead. Not that I could ever really forget the Christmas season of the prior year, at least not one lesson it so graciously provided.

John and I had written a Christmas newsletter back in 1995 and perhaps prematurely disclosed that I was off of the "terminal" list. The response was gratifying, nonetheless, as many of those close to us openly discussed my good fortune. Some said they had been afraid to ask how I was doing for fear I might be on the proverbial deathbed or even worse. Some had been working very hard to rein in their own fear not just of cancer but of the debilitating treatment options as well. We were far from being alone as these folks had been vicariously experiencing our anxiety and had felt our relief. In fact, several had taken a great interest in my natural therapy and one in particular referred a friend with cancer to learn of my experiences. And now in December of 1996, we knew a number of people on shark cartilage for cancer and/or arthritis and those who took the concept seriously seemed to have benefited from it.

One woman named Marilyn Bollinger, who is also a member of the GYN support group I had been attending for something like a year and a half by this time, was especially aggressive in seeking complementary treatments. She went through just one series of chemotherapy to bring her Stage III ovarian cancer under control. Not one to sit idly by, she exhaustively questioned John and me about the cartilage therapy and almost immediately went on it adjusting the dosage as needed to keep her CA-125 tumor markers down. At the same time she pursued other alternative approaches very diligently.

She plotted her treatment course not only by researching her condition immediately but by also establishing rapport with her oncologist (the same as mine) and using his able assistance along with that of other health professionals to expand and evaluate her treatment program. Consequently, she was in the enviable position of being able to smoothly make use of conventional modalities should the need arise. To this day, John and I are painfully aware of our mistake in not being similarly prompt and aggressive. This is the principal reason for writing this book. Had we not gotten busy when we did, I would not have been here to write anything.

Since this time, I noted others who had contracted cancer but were more attuned from the very beginning to alternative approaches and did not have to start from behind in fighting the disease. Such people are especially fortunate.

chapter fourteen

Fine Tuning for Life

The usual six- or seven-day wait following a blood draw to learn the CA-125 tumor marker was never a comfortable time and in 1997 I faced eight of these intervals, the last one as unsettling as the first. Parachutists sometimes say their third jump was the most frightening but that subsequent leaps became progressively easier. My case might have also shown an improving anxiety pattern except for feeling blindfolded. Upon "landing," each tumor marker opened up as a heart-stopping surprise.

On January 15, when my latest marker of only 12.4 was revealed, I trembled but only momentarily as the marker's benign significance rapidly sank in. My nerves were further soothed as my oncologist repeated aloud the changes made in my regimen. "Your marker had been between 46 and 95 for eight or nine months," he said, thoughtfully, "then you increased your daily shark cartilage dosage by about 70 percent and we get this!" My oncologist tapped and pointed his finger almost reverently at the 12.4 marker now recorded on my medical records. My primary care internist in an office visit just two days before had responded in a similar way without yet knowing of this latest very favorable result but again called me "the miracle woman" based on the previous 37.2 marker.

Both of the doctors seemed pleased with my weight level of 150 pounds and seemed impressed by my tumor marker response to the increased cartilage intake. As one would expect, my oncologist especially appeared very interested in keeping up with the latest cartilage research.

* * * *

Although the future would hold many more surprises, at this point in my recovery I had confidence in the course chosen. Yet it is impossible to explain, at least with any degree of reasonableness, why dark apprehension followed each CA-125 blood draw. Perhaps it was because I was painfully aware from all of the conversations I had had with other seriously ill patients, that most would face what is characterized in the athletic arena as "the agony of defeat." And, indeed, on several occasions hopelessness had attacked me and I experienced a considerable measure of that agony. The dark apprehension spoken of, then, may have been the distant echoes from those I had known who had lost all in their struggle against death.

As with their pharmaceutical counterparts, natural cancer remedies have significant failure rates – enough deaths, in fact, to enable critics to gloss over the many apparent successes. If a natural substance happens to produce a five percent positive response rate, actually proving this by even the most sophisticated testing procedure would be next to impossible because a margin of error is always present. However, unlike most pharmaceuticals, natural substances seldom produce serious side effects and several can be used simultaneously to enhance overall effectiveness. But the reductionist outlook of conventional medicine invariably precludes the testing of such combinations. This proclivity to isolate the healing element of a single substance, of course, favors the stronger but harsher pharmaceuticals. However, high grade shark cartilage which has sometimes shown an effectiveness level of 50 percent or more for certain tumors, including the deadly ovarian variety, is now being "officially" tested as a whole and natural product. But again, can government bureaucrats be trusted? As always, there is no escaping that question.

The official United States outlook toward cancer came under at first naive and then insightful, scorching scrutiny in the 1995 documentary film, "The Politics of Cancer." Its smallish subtitle, "(a study in chaos)," though in parentheses and without capitalization did prepare one for the viewing but not fully. We had heard about the film and its noted Polish-born director, Andrzej Krakowski, and had decided to see it but could find no nearby theater listing. Consequently, a couple of years after its release, John was able to buy a video copy put out by Healing Arts Documentary Productions, Inc. and by 1997 we had watched it more than once.

In at least one way, Krakowski's early life paralleled that of Stanislaw Burzynski, M.D., the beleaguered medical maverick and humanitarian of Texas mentioned earlier. Both were forced out of their native Poland by communist excesses only to face something akin to dictatorial excesses in the United States. Apparently, Krakowski's family had been blacklisted by Communist authorities in Poland because of Jewish blood and political indifference.

Having to refine his self-described "atrocious" English hardly interfered with Krakowski's film making ability as he is credited with such works as "Eminent Domain" with Donald Sutherland and "Triumph of the Spirit" with Willem Dafoe. "The Politics of Cancer" had played at the Cannes Film Festival in May of 1995 and probably would have gone on to win any number of awards except for its somber subject matter.

Krakowski's wife, Elizabeth, was diagnosed in 1989 with breast cancer and the documentary highlights her responses to the treatment program. Elizabeth Krakowski, a microbiologist, might also have had the full benefit of alternative approaches had the political and economic cross currents been less severe. And despite husband Andrzej traveling to Cuba with the leading shark cartilage researcher, I. William Lane, and finding former terminal patients doing well, such knowledge wasn't enough. The film's final segment finds a doctor telling Elizabeth that her metastatic cancer is in remission only to be followed by images of her funeral six months later, 1994.

The film no doubt reflected its maker's later apprehension and agony as it progressed from a rather quiet tempo into a thunderous, penetrating storm. No overall narration was used to tie the numerous interview segments together and a great number of people – politicos, bureaucrats, doctors and cancer victims alike – were interviewed to better fulfill the film's central mission. Perhaps this resulted in the lack of particulars on the wife's very sudden and tragic death. And perhaps because of this omission, the documentary is all the more haunting and unforgettable.

As a child in Warsaw, Krakowski remembered hearing of a family friend living in the United States returning to Russia to treat his cancer. Later, Andrzej asked why, and his father replied that given time he would understand the reason. And now Andrzej does understand and he vowed that should he contract cancer, he would not opt for conventional treatments.

This information about Andrzej Krakowski was discussed in a telephone conversation with the distributor and was included with the video in the form of written documents. John later discussed this case with researcher Dr. I. William Lane and it was his understanding that the wife, Elizabeth, had started taking the shark cartilage when it was far too late for it to be effective.

Here are more of the film maker's reported conclusions: traditional cancer treatment modalities have changed little since the 1950's; that there is a blanket of fatalism confronting cancer patients that doesn't exist in other countries such as Germany, Poland and Cuba; that the power centers in this country may not want to find a cancer cure as there would be more people on social security and pensions; that power brokers are not likely to say this country has been going in the wrong direction in cancer research as it would be political suicide; that one goal of many physicians and hospitals is to hew the line of conventionality to avoid lawsuits; and, finally, that government bureaucrats are often indifferent or hostile toward promising treatments. Under present circumstances, Krakowski suggested that cancer patients do the homework necessary to wisely take charge of their own treatments.

* * * *

John and I are now much more aware of wayward political and economic currents following my cancer-related experiences and our conclusions now parallel those of film maker Andrzej Krakowski. But it can't be stressed strongly enough just how close I came to becoming a statistic and had government edict required I wait for two or six weeks for a "compassionate use" permit to obtain the shark cartilage powder, it would have sealed my fate. And John and I are also acutely aware that my success with shark cartilage is officially counted as a success for the therapeutic poisons which nearly killed me. When government lies, it lies big!

Andrzej Krakowski did note modern medicine's tendency to indeed keep an eye on the bottom line and was fully aware of the troubling role of modern HMOs, but he did not seem to emphasize the role of the pharmaceutical cartel. Of course, my husband had some training in economics and this no doubt contributed to his being fully aware of its role in shaping political policy. But as always, John is just plain John.

And John did grumble in mid January of '97. When I took it upon myself to phase out the retention enemas in favor of the oral doses. And he nearly bumped the ceiling when I lowered the daily intake from 100 plus grams of the cartilage powder to a more livable 70 grams. When the February 7 blood draw showed my CA-125 tumor marker had marched from 12.4 right back up to 35.5, John actually bumped the ceiling. No matter, I was asserting myself and my intuition was telling me to stop worrying so much and I cut the daily dosage level back again to about 66 grams. And when my marker of March 18 came down eight points to 27.1, I responded, "See-e-e" with as much authority as my lean voice could muster.

My male oncologist had earlier suggested I might find a lower dosage satisfactory for a maintenance level but that was not the reason for my new effort at independence. It was all the men, including my husband, who had surrounded me with advice. But, alas, my push to assert myself was tempered by a serious cough, sore throat and fever and I found myself once again dependent on the comforting care of my chauvinistic husband. And I decided, then and there, the prospects for more rebellion were actually quite dim.

* * * *

"But then, who knows?" might have been added to that final lament as I soon recovered. Every little tickle and cough, nevertheless, I still felt was somehow connected to the malignancy. And these little recoveries, therefore, loomed as happy events. But more gratifying was my continued improvement in health and for the remainder of 1997 it was not necessary to resort to the very high cartilage dosages of months earlier. This is not to say that John didn't fret and try to convince me otherwise as his worry was perennial. But I did do some fine tuning.

On April 29, my tumor marker bounced up a little from 27.1 to 30.6 even though my daily cartilage intake remained about the same at nearly 68 grams. John became very nervous about this rise and checked his mathematical calculations on the dosage level again and again and tried to convince me to "listen to reason," but again I stood my ground and continued the same level of cartilage ingestion. And even though my daily cartilage intake did slip very slightly to just over 66 grams, my marker for June 3 had dropped over 8 points to 22.0, a very satisfying result, indeed, especially considering that I had dropped the shark liver oil capsules and some of the enzymes from my regimen some weeks before. And despite having had some strange "traveling" aches in my bones and joints for several months, I was confident enough to do some more fine tuning.

My tumor marker of July 15 had moved up only slightly, to 23. 0, and was still within the "safe" range below 35. Therefore, I felt safe lowering my daily cartilage intake to just below 60 grams, about five or six grams below what I had been taking. John was still upset about my "taking unnecessary chances" and when my next marker jumped up, so did he. On September 16, the marker had registered 35.9 and John's overwrought response did have its effect as I promptly brought the daily dosage back up some six grams to its previous level. This move did calm John some but a little later he truly became unsettled – as did I.

On Saturday, September 27, we had been in Tucson shopping and were settled in at a restaurant for a mid afternoon lunch when John pointed to my right eye. The socket was both swollen and painful and the eye was watery and sensitive to light. The condition had been progressing for several days but was accorded little thought as it was similar to my past episodes of inflammation. When I told John that I would take care of it at home, he protested and we drove directly to Urgent Care. And, indeed, another mystery! No cause could be found, not even by my ophthalmologist three days later. Although I had been administered Prednisolone Sodium Phosphate at Urgent Care and continued the eye drops at home, my eye had nearly swollen shut before the condition improved and vanished.

* * * *

Although 1997 saw a return of some of the old ailments, my digestive problems had improved markedly. Furthermore, for the first time since my cancer diagnosis, I was adjusting quite nicely to my daily health regimen which I knew was most likely permanent. And since the marker of November 18, 1997, the year's last, dropped only fractionally, from 35.9 to 35.7, I responded to John's concern and increased my daily cartilage dosage just a little. And even our dog's eating propensities taught us a little lesson.

John likes trees and, consequently, our rural home has perhaps 120 of them (he tried counting the scattered trees several times but came up with different answers). The one apricot tree, two or three years back, had a very fruitful season and we were astounded by the little dog's reaction. Although we also own dwarf peach trees and had observed her occasionally breaking the seed shells and eating the kernels, the dog seemed to favor eating the equally hard apricot seeds.

Of course, we were in competition with the birds who ate the apricot flesh. We had so many apricots that we picked only those easily reached and a great number of seeds pecked clean by the birds soon covered the ground – and this is when our little dog started cracking the shells in earnest. In fact, she had hidden some seeds to be eaten months later. And that is when we wondered why this little creature appeared so needful of the kernels. I tasted one and it seemed quite bitter but guessed that a dog's taste buds were different. Naturally, John could hardly accept such an uninvolved explanation and went on to talk about "the whispers within."

Over the vast eons, living creatures were forced to make choices which sometimes had survival value that over succeeding generations evolved into instinctual predispositions. And according to John, we were witnessing such behavior here. Our cute cocker spaniel mix was heeding dark, primordial "whispers" prompting her to eat these kernels. Now, this made perfect sense to John but I told him that I wasn't about to eat the kernels because unlike the dog I knew they released poisonous cyanide during digestion. Besides, the whispers I heard were telling me not to listen to him.

In time, I did check our reference materials and learned that the apricot kernels were a nutritious food and safe in limited quantities. And we had noted that our dog usually ate but one or two kernels at a time. The product laetrile is derived mainly from apricot kernels and while it has been put down as useless by government bureaucrats, the basic substance has been found in more than a thousand plants. In fact, people unknowingly ingest it by eating such foods as lima beans, cashews, and brown rice. This substance, amygdalin, is also called vitamin B17 and is also contained in peach seed kernels and the bitter almond but the naturally occurring cyanide associated with the apricot kernel is thought to enhance its cancer fighting potential.

Although positive results have been reported using laetrile coupled with certain digestive enzymes, a wholesome diet, and vitamins and minerals, especially vitamin A, I resisted John's efforts to add the low-cost apricot kernels to my diet. All the poisons used in my chemotherapy caused me to worry about even normally benign and naturally occurring forms such as the awful sounding cyanide variety associated with apricot kernels. We knew that an average-sized adult could safely take up to six kernels per hour up to 30 per day but I refused to even take one per day. Of course, John had to show my fears were baseless by taking a modest amount himself, about 12 kernels per day divided evenly between breakfast and dinner.

John suggested I watch to see if he keeled over or suffered the dizziness, blurred vision, and nausea associated with cyanide poisoning and, of course, he suffered none of these things. And, after about three months, I took just one kernel per day plus a very small amount ground up and sprinkled as spice on certain dishes. At first, we used our own apricot kernels but later found a source that sold the shelled kernels in two-pound bags and recommended it as a wholesome spice to be ground up in small amounts as needed. But John didn't mind slowly eating the whole kernels with a meal and in time neither did I and increased my daily consumption to five kernels during breakfast and five at dinner. Now, I look back and wonder what all the fuss was about and if it helps my condition even a smidgen, it is worth it because it is both inexpensive and easy to take.

As it has been used since ancient times as a wholesome food and an aid in controlling cancer, today's bureaucratic attacks against the apricot kernel though harsh and loud are so hollow that even our little dog knows better. It is interesting that the more nature-bound communities still in existence whose members seldom contract cancer and who live long and healthfully in a meager environment have one characteristic in common: they allow little food to go to waste, including apricot kernels which they often store and eat on a regular basis. Another little echo of our dog's behavior.

* * * *

In the year 1997, there was something that both John and I found troubling. We had heard from those familiar with our nation's criminal injustice system (no misspelling here) that we were taking risks talking about my cancer experiences even on an informal basis. And we know of one elderly charity volunteer who was sued for more than a quarter million dollars by an author (with three lawyers) partly because the volunteer lacked the means to fully defend herself. Her "crime" was making a mistake in listing one of the author's books!

Another disturbing experience involved John and the cancer clinic library that patients and others alike are encouraged to visit as it features potentially life saving publications and videos. Of course, it consists primarily of promotional materials provided by pharmaceutical companies and other conventional sources. But in the back near a conspicuous disclaimer are unconventional materials primarily concerned with nutritional and other health issues which only obliquely compete with the wealthy pharmaceutical cartel. Although technically a nutritional supplement, shark cartilage does compete more directly with the cartel as clinical trials and anecdotal evidence have shown it frequently effective in controlling several types of chronic conditions especially those involving cancerous, fast-growing solid tumors. Thus, would shark cartilage books and videos be treated more coolly?

John and I would soon find out as we had earlier donated an item or two to the small library and finally we donated the two books on shark cartilage therapy written by Dr. I. William Lane and Linda Comac. A short time later when John tried to include the companion video, "Shark Cartilage: A Promise Kept," the library person we had spoken to previously now appeared almost hostile suggesting that some clinic doctors objected to the materials. Even though it was obvious he was now persona non grata, John explained, among other things, that the video included the latest reports of clinical trials and other information that might be critical especially for terminally ill patients who want to include shark cartilage in their diets. Then John said, "Here," and held the video out to her. Although she took it and it later appeared on the library shelf, it was obvious that censorship existed here.

To be sure, there are few genuine resources available for the seriously ill cancer patient for whom conventional therapies have failed. But the challenges are even greater for those who can't start conventional treatments because none had been shown effective for the particular cancer involved and, thus, time becomes all the more crucial. This was especially evident when a neighbor's sister was diagnosed with a particularly fast growing and virulent form of pancreatic cancer and was told there was absolutely no valid treatment available. The family had close European roots and knew this was probably untrue but everyone felt so rushed and confused that by the time an alternative option was selected, it was far too late. We were to learn later that this very deadly kind of cancer can indeed be successfully treated. Because a pancreatic malignancy typically grows fast, immediately ingesting massive doses of high grade shark cartilage is an especially promising avenue to slow, halt or even reverse the progression of this horrible disease. And although there is some compelling anecdotal evidence supporting this, such information is not likely to be on the shelf either at the library or the book store – or any other place, for that matter.

Not only is there a lack of readily available information for the terminally ill cancer patient, but John and I are convinced that there are "authorities" who muddy the water by pretending to be objective purveyors of alternative information and advice. It is one thing for a so-called authority to speak out of ignorance and something else to mislead the seriously ill for personal gain. More than once, John and I have heard or read that it is impossible for the body to absorb the bioactive macro proteins of shark cartilage and thus impossible for it to help control cancer. These prevaricators certainly haven't convinced my body of this, but some terminal patients may have thus been denied a chance to live. In a lighter vein, my husband told me he had some ideas on the matter but instead turned to yet another crazy notion, his most incredible yet.

* * * *

To my astonishment, John wanted to style my hair for "an exquisite fashion statement to rival that of a goddess." He had watched – perhaps for the first time – as my hair dresser cut, snipped, combed and styled my hair with high drama, standing back and appraising the work at certain points to make sure it was done just right. And her flourishes prevailed as the outcome was so beautiful that even John noticed. Then out of the blue I heard, "I bet I could do that." "No way," said I, "Go cut your own hair." (Actually, John does cut his own hair and botches it every time. I trim only the back. You see, he is bald and combs his hair over and forward and calls the dubious result, "The great cover-up.")

Actually, after months of being pestered, I gave in – at least to some extent – but that's a subject for the next chapter as I did manage to hold off the inevitable until the middle of 1998, the year of a new beginning.

chapter fifteen

A New Beginning in an Old Flavor

The year, 1998 was similar to the year of my brain surgery, 1995, as it, too, was to see critical surgery. But this time it was John's turn as he suffered a ruptured appendix, no less. And his full-cut surgery was all the more serious because of his old age, 68 years to be exact.

The Christmas holiday season of 1997-98 did augur well, at least for me, as we had traveled to Prescott, Arizona for a family gathering as we had exactly three years earlier and this time I felt much better despite the extreme cold and blustery snowfall. Although I contracted the flu which had been prevalent, my tumor marker of January 13 was down from the 35.7 of nearly two months earlier to a more satisfying 27.1 – this drop coming despite my increasing the daily cartilage intake by only one gram to 67, considerably less than intended.

There were times I thought such preciseness in calculating my daily dosage was extreme, but I now knew better. In this instance, the daily average per one-pound (454-gram) cartilage container ranged from 62.4 to 72.8 grams and I was aiming for a consistent 70. As can be seen, the spread between the lowest and highest container average was more than 10 grams and it must be remembered that my "calculating" husband was keeping track of this and, thus, I received repeated and timely feedback. Had I relied only on vague impressions of the amount of powder taken, who knows what the end result might have been. Also, there were distractions.

During my flu episode just mentioned, I might have become distracted and reduced my cartilage intake had I not been fully alert. Toward the middle of February my left eye socket took its cue from the right side and now months later became sore and swollen plus the eye itself more light sensitive. This repeat of the mysterious condition was extremely distracting and in the trouble-some days before it, too, finally vanished, I also might have skipped some doses had I lowered my guard. And the need to carefully heed the exacting requirements of the cartilage regimen became all the more evident when I apparently achieved a surprising out-come from yet another "minor" adjustment.

* * * *

It seemed unlikely that I would be able to ingest fewer than 65 grams of the cartilage powder daily and still maintain a com-fortable CA-125 tumor marker at or below 35. Consequently, I made up my mind to maintain at least this level daily for the fore-seeable future. In January, moreover, I realized that I seldom noted the time between an oral dose and the start of a meal. And my 40- or 45-minute estimates of the intervening time may have been erroneous and the actual intervals far shorter.

Taking a cue from John's tendency to keep a precise record of everything numerical, I now began setting the kitchen timer (which John, of course, had checked for accuracy) for 45 minutes so that the interval would be at least this long thus allowing the cartilage/liquid mix to quickly pass through my empty stomach and its destructive acids. We were aware that cartilage research-ers had begun recommending an hour interval but had never taken it that seriously because of being used to the earlier recommenda-tions which were shorter. But what a difference a carefully timed interval apparently makes as my tumor marker of April 7, 1998, following no change in the dosage level, was now down more than nine points to 18.7 – and was another great relief following John's emergency appendectomy!

Not mentioned, his emergency in at least one respect was similar to that surrounding my surgery in 1995 to remove, what was later determined, a dead, but still dangerous, brain tumor. John's surgical preparations were also rushed for fear the appendix would burst and threaten his life. Despite this urgent response, it apparently ruptured at the very last minute. Nevertheless, after a very tense and painful postoperative week, he came home not that much worse for wear. Curiously, John's urgent operation took place on March 25 – the same month and day as my emergency brain surgery three years before!

* * * *

Curious coincidences had already been noted especially that of John coming across the date of poor Barney's apparent suicide etched on a steel support in a cancer clinic rest room. Half jokingly, I suggested high portent in this latest coincidence saying that the powers on Mount Olympus were telling him something and that he had better watch out (John seems to have an affinity for matters ancient). As expected, he suggested the two events were coincident and nothing more.

But there was more, said I, and in trying to appeal to the scientific side, asked my dear hubby what the chances were of the two urgent surgeries falling on the same day and month within just three years. But before he answered, I reminded him that he had just stumbled across a remote epitaph and had found it singularly intriguing: "Together we walked... Together we died." I suggested again that these powers from on high were grappling with his insurgence and he had better heed these revelations, obscure though they may be.

He then proceeded to give me a lesson in statistics, ending it with the notion that it was all coincidental and nothing more. But when I reminded him this is exactly what critics of my natural therapy say about the positive results obtained, he remained quiet for just a spell. "You have to allow for that one-in-a-thousand long shot," said he. John!!

* * * *

Now I knew, all this was inexplicable by chance except for an insignificant speck, according to he who calculates and measures and is forever dealing in probabilities. But when the oncology nurse made an impromptu telephone call to report the results of my May 26 blood draw, the emotion in her voice told it all: this tiny bit of uncertainty had been wiped away. My CA-125 tumor marker was now down to 2.5, certainly the lowest I had ever heard of and from the repeated suggestions by the nurse on how very positive this marker was, it was something novel in her experience as well.

There was also some very satisfying news on the canine front which was hardly less stellar, at least from our little dog's point of view. For months she had been favoring one hind leg or the other perhaps caused, we thought, by stepping on thorny goathead seedpods. Early rains had produced an abundance of these noxious seeds and since she was only seven years old we didn't seriously consider osteoarthritis. But our veterinarian diagnosed it when the dog's locomotion came to a virtual halt and, strangely, she often became constipated. He explained the osteoarthritic pain had actually impeded positioning to evacuate!

Our veterinarian outlined two therapy choices: the first, he said, was based on "good science," but is only a palliative treatment of aspirin; the second involves administering a combination basically of chondroitin sulfate, glucosamine and sometimes a cartilage powder. He said this natural combination based on what some call "junk science" not only has been shown to reduce arthritic pain but appears to promote joint healing as well. Needless to say, we chose to administer this natural combination – and for good reason.

Not only had my rheumatoid arthritis been tamed within days by the massive ingestion of shark cartilage but husband John had similarly rid his knees of osteoarthritis, although the standard dosage of bovine cartilage he used took four months. Despite our favorable experiences, I was a bit concerned, when John added one-half the human dosage of bovine cartilage to the standard dosage of the glucosamine-chondroitin combination already supplied by the veterinarian. But within five or six days, our little dog was moving about and within 14 days was up and running full tilt! Obviously, I needn't have worried about the extra cartilage dosage as there were no discernible side effects, whatsocver. Moreover, we were able to cut out the extra cartilage and halve the veterinarian's combined glucosamine dosage and "Coco" continued to do just fine.

Interestingly, glucosamine is derived from the chitin of crab shells and chondroitin sulfate from bovine cartilage. Sometimes pure shark, bovine and/or porcine cartilage as well as other ingredients are added to this combination. It could hardly be argued that our dog's response to this therapy was due to the placebo effect as it is impossible to communicate one's expectation of outcome to an animal – at least, not with any level of precision. This independent curb of the placebo effect is particularly germane since the previously mentioned clinical trials and more recent anecdotal outcomes show positive responses in treating not only animal arthritis but such cancer as well using shark cartilage alone.

* * * *

Following John's appendectomy, my cartilage-controlled rheumatoid arthritis symptoms returned and though less severe, started disturbing my sleep. Strangely, just one knuckle of my right index finger became swollen the way most of my knuckles had before starting the shark cartilage therapy back in 1994. Except for the swelling of this lone outer knuckle, the return of my old arthritic pain was not unexpected since I had to help with heavy lifting during John's convalescence. But the pain continued even after John resumed the heavy chores and I decided what was good for "Coco" might be good for me. Of course, there is no telling whether the cartilage would have fully tamed my arthritis again, yet my ingesting a glucosamine-chondroitin combination did quickly result in pain relief. The lone knuckle remained swollen, however.

During this hectic period, John got to style my hair – actually, just the back portion – as I hadn't time for my hairdresser and was desperate for an interim trim. John made all sorts of "stylistic" promises, but only uttered a series of "Oops" once the clipping started. He ended with a dramatic flourish and a loud, "Oh-oh" and I was afraid to look. But upon adjusting the double mirrors, I was pleasantly surprised. John claimed it was a stylistic masterpiece, but I sighed in relief as it was adequate, though barely. I decided to say nothing and let John dream of being a high-fashion hair stylist and vowed never again as all the fuss and uncertainty wasn't worth it. He can keep his "Oops" and "Oh-oh's" and trim his own hair!

* * * *

When our phone rang one day in July of 1998, the deep, thunderous voice on the other end sounded like that of Barney (who, remember, had apparently committed suicide three years earlier) but John had only a momentary start as the more commanding tones of this voice became apparent. It was that of Dante Ruccio, N.D.C., a naturopathic consultant from Newark, New Jersey. His research effort on the use of shark cartilage to control cancer had been noted in the 1993 reference volume entitled, *Alternative Medicine: the Definitive Guide*, compiled by The Burton Goldberg Group. Needless to say, we were surprised to hear from this well-known doctor of naturopathy.

Dr. Ruccio had been informed of my book-writing effort and seemed concerned that John and I might be unaware of the routine suppression of nontoxic cancer therapies by the conventional pharmaceutical interests. It took John only a minute or two to convince him that we had become fully aware of this on our own and that we understood as well how the mainstream media especially has been influenced by the huge budgets set aside for pharmaceutical advertising. With this out of the way, the conversation turned to other matters.

The doctor first opined that scientist Judah Folkman's newly developed drugs, angiostatin and endostatin, which worked so well on mice, are likely to work on humans as well. Even though they work essentially the same way shark cartilage does by cutting off the blood supply to malignant tumors, unlike cartilage they are patentable as conventional drugs and will likely produce huge profits. He only regretted shark cartilage wasn't used more as an interim measure to save more lives. Ruccio said there are a number of other natural substances available to help fight cancer but in his experience none works as well as shark cartilage. (Interestingly, he was apparently the first U.S. doctor to also observe the Swiss cheese character of cartilage-treated tumors).

It should be mentioned that Dr. Ruccio was involved in a clinical trial cited in the 1993 reference volume just mentioned. Ninety-four seriously ill cancer patients took high levels of premium grade shark cartilage as a supplement and 12 of these patients went into complete remission and except for two, the remaining number received varying degrees of benefit. Now, Dr. Ruccio estimated that he had counseled an additional 2,000 mostly late-stage cancer victims in the use of cartilage. It was obvious that the good doctor was highly enthusiastic about his work virtually exploding with information, much of it very technical. And a number of his clinical observations on cartilage therapy do bear relating.

When cartilage antiangiogenesis causes a tumor to disintegrate, he observed, the tumor marker may rise, often abruptly, causing the patient considerable consternation. (This is exactly what happened to me, especially at the start of my cartilage therapy!)

The doctor also observed that a tumor will actually expand during dissolution if the blood blockage occurs on the return side and increases its internal pressure. (Years earlier, a woman on cartilage said one tumor expanded for a time while her others shrank!)

Interestingly, his observations revealed not only no harm occurred from the use of shark cartilage immediately before and following major surgery, but that it may have actually aided the healing. (I had stopped the shark cartilage regimen only days before my major brain surgery and yet healing was fast and complete!)

Although conventional wisdom suggests that shark cartilage will only work on solid tumors – carcinomas and sarcomas – Ruccio has observed some beneficial results on non-solid cancers, such as leukemia and lymphoma. (I have only heard of distant reports of this happening but the cartilage may also boost the immune system in subtle ways.)

The doctor emphasized that it could be taken not only by retention enema but orally as well as long as the stomach is empty and each dosage is taken at least an hour before mealtime. He recommended mixing each oral dose fresh with eight ounces of icy water for improved taste and greater solubility. He often recommends that one start by thus drinking 24-gram doses of the cartilage four times daily (96 grams) spread throughout day.

While Ruccio feels the excision of tumors is usually beneficial, the outcome of radiation or chemotherapy is usually less so. In fact, he said the true deadliness of these treatment modalities is concealed by attending physicians ascribing the primary cause of death not specifically to the chemotherapy or radiation but to secondary complications such as pneumonia or organ failure. (As already mentioned, the partial failure of my digestive organs from the chemotherapy finally came very close to doing me in and I am reasonably sure had I died the specific cause of death, namely, chemotherapy, would not have been "officially" recorded.)

All in all, John and I had the distinct feeling we had made contact with a highly motivated researcher who was in the field for the good he could do (he charges cancer victims no consultation fee!) This was the first time a major researcher took the time to call us about my experiences and to explore ways to get the message out to terminal cancer victims that alternate avenues for possible recovery exist now. Some might find him blunt and obsessed with his work, but we found him inspiring. Actually, his sincere interest increased our desire to attend the upcoming 1998 Cancer Control Society conference in Pasadena, California.

* * * *

Before leaving for the Labor Day weekend cancer convention, we did see my oncologist August 6 who told us that my blood draw of nine days earlier registered a CA-125 tumor marker of 5.0, only a small rise from the previous 2.5 marker. I had made a slight change in my cartilage regimen by not taking the day's final dosage at bedtime but an hour earlier so that I could have a light snack before retiring, but I could sense my doctor felt the increase was an inconsequential blip and he simply waved it off. In fact, his attitude seemed to parallel that of my primary care doctor just weeks earlier in suggesting there was little else for him to do but monitor my condition and have me come in for periodic checkups. My primary care internist did have me report for a CT scan and, happily, it showed no regrowth of the brain tumor which had been removed three years earlier.

With all this good news there was one unsettling event, however. A publicist planning a health story for a local television station had contacted me about my survival efforts using non-pharmaceutical approaches, particularly shark cartilage and asked if I was willing to participate in the program. Although I was aware that TV networks sometimes give the most negative spin possible in their reports on nontoxic therapies, I answered yes. The publicist telephoned me several times and though my naturopathic physician immediately returned his call, my oncologist and primary care physicians apparently declined to respond. Since this avenue was unresponsive, the producer tried to highlight my support group for the story but those in charge of the group declined because I would be interviewed and would thus discuss my positive experiences using the shark cartilage supplement!!! It was feared that the support group would thereby be associated with the natural shark cartilage therapy.

In the March 1998 issue of Dr. Julian Whitaker's "Health & Healing" newsletter, this well-known medical doctor and book author wrote that the pharmaceutical industry practically underwrites not only the business of medicine but medical education as well – and this promotion equates to an expenditure per doctor of $13,000 yearly!

Needless to say, all honest doctors are under a great deal of pressure and must proceed warily. Even this nation's courts are not immune to the pressures exerted by those who hold the powerful dollar, as exemplified by the experience of William D. Kelley, D.D.S., whose nontoxic nutritional plan I now largely adhere to, as mentioned. Decades ago he was ordered by a federal judge not to write or otherwise tell of his cancer experiences and treatment protocol again!!! It's little wonder, then, that stories which put natural therapies in a negative light get such big headlines. Who would have ever thought my positive experiences with cartilage therapy was worthy of censorship! But this journey of mine continues.

* * * *

Again our journey to the three-day Annual Cancer Control Society Convention in Pasadena, California was well worth the travel. One of the speakers was shark cartilage researcher, Dr. I. William Lane, who not only updated the conference on the latest cartilage research, but also helped another internationally recognized immunology researcher, Egyptian-born Mamdooh Ghoneum, Ph.D., introduce a new, clinically tested product called, MGN-3. **Seven published efficacy studies involving a total of 72 patients, had shown this natural immune complex to triple natural killer (NK) protection and enhance B-cell and T-cell activity.** While this product, distributed by Lane Labs-USA, Inc., may be taken alone, Dr. Lane also suggested that it was a natural adjunct to shark cartilage therapy. In closing, Dr. Lane not only announced a new book of his would appear soon, but that news of a new and dramatic breakthrough was in the offing.

Ralph W. Moss, Ph.D., the author of the highly acclaimed exposé, *The Cancer Industry*, spoke on suppressed nontoxic cancer treatments. This noted critic of the U.S. monolithic medical system also authored a number of other books and documents, including the award-winning PBS documentary, "The Cancer War." Thus, especial interest was shown here in his refusal two decades ago to abide Sloan-Kettering's disregard of certain laetrile research findings that catapulted him out of the conventional domain and into an abiding interest of alternative cancer treatments. Nevertheless, it was the story of a teenage boy running from home to escape chemotherapy, and an impassioned plea for medical freedom by a cancer survivor's husband that hit closest to home.

* * * *

Mary Jo Siegel had sought treatment for her non-Hodgkin's lymphoma from Stanislaw Burzynski, M.D., and she credits the much persecuted doctor with saving her life without causing ill side effects. Her husband, Steve, told how FDA bureaucrats threatened Dr. Burzynski with possible life in prison for actually following the Hippocratic Oath even though not one of his many patients had filed a complaint against him!! Even though government prosecutors with their fabricated charges lost in court, the harassment of the doctor and his largely late-stage cancer patients continues.

Consequently, Siegel fervently admonished all to become proactive in pushing for legislation giving more control of health decisions to the adult patient even if the patient decides to use now officially discouraged nontoxic modalities. His thesis? Excessive government intrusion doesn't make for better medical care.

One government test method was especially troubling to Siegel as it involved establishing a test protocol more appropriate for harsh pharmaceuticals, not slower acting nontoxic substances such as Burzynski's antineoplastons. Clinical cases which show less than a 50 percent tumor reduction over a stipulated period, he explained, are classed as failures. This distorts the data so it really shouldn't surprise anyone that a person with, say, a 44 percent tumor shrinkage over an arbitrary period might do very well and be much better off in the long run. In fact, this was the actual experience of one Burzynski patient now doing quite nicely.

At age 16, Billy Best, as you might remember, found himself faced with a harsh dilemma: run away from home or face more chemotherapy for his Hodgkin's disease, another form of lymphatic cancer. Naturally, he chose the former to escape the latter by pawning some his worldly possessions and hopping a bus for Houston. Having taken along his prized skateboard, he found kindred souls with whom to skate and blend in. Televised pleas of his mother quickly convinced him to return home. Now, after a three-year hiatus he stood here on the same dais again very tall and straight speaking before this 1998 Cancer Control Society conference.

Much matured in three years, he spoke eloquently of his experience and plans to enter medical school to be an alternative doctor and give the kind of help he had received. Sadly, Billy recounted how one man who helped guide him – as well as others – toward the nontoxic compound 714X and Essiac herbal tea (which checkups confirmed had likely eliminated the lymphoma), was given a rather lengthy prison sentence. Now in radiant health, Billy seemed keenly appreciative of this man and others who had helped him. Even more sadly, now 20-year-old Billy realized he might have been snatched from home by state authorities – all because he sought an alternative path to escape the devastation of yet more chemotherapy!

Interestingly, we saw him with his mother, Susan, at a booth, as distributors of the Essiac herbal tea that's so familiar to them. Significantly, Susan Best observed that alternative advocates who exercise the First Amendment right are the ones often thrown in prison. "It's not the quiet, ordinary person they are after," she concluded.

"Woof"

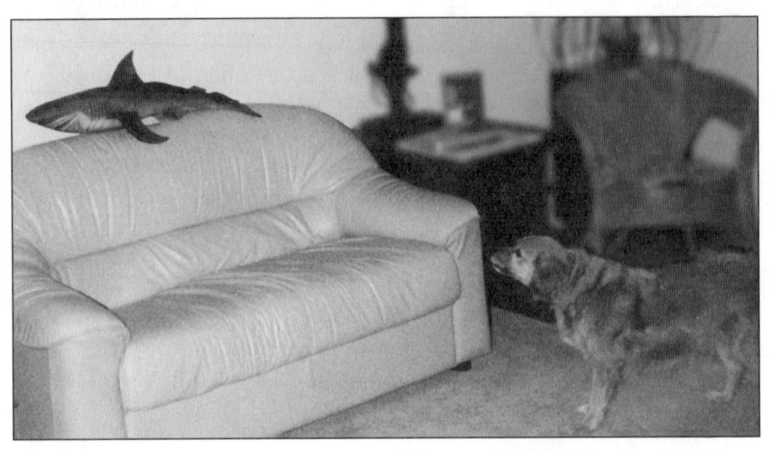

Upon spotting our newly acquired shark-formed pillow, our little spaniel mix immediately – and easily – leapt back and assumed a defensive posture punctuated with appropriate growls and "woofs."

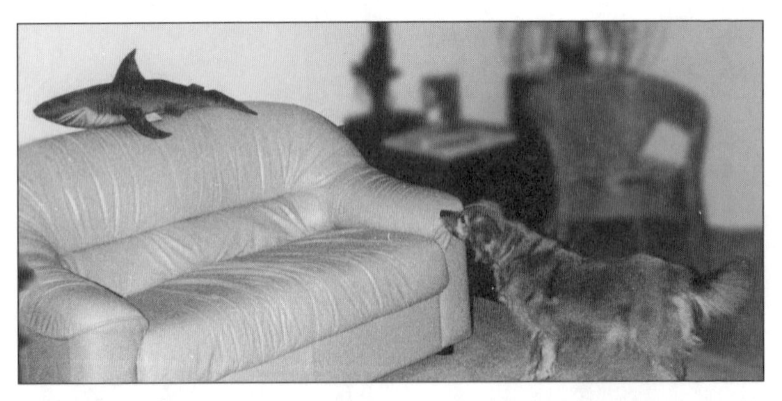

Starting from a prudent distance, she bravely confronts her potential adversary – her once arthritic hind legs holding up splendidly.

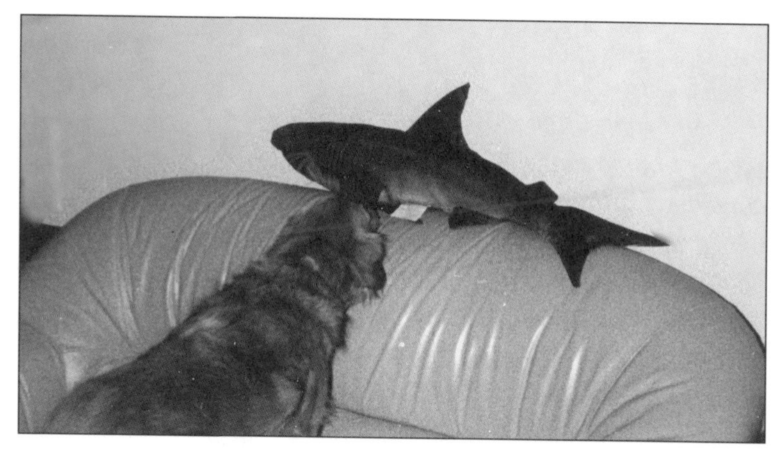

It took some minutes of noisy but cautious sniffing before she was satisfied that all was safe – safe enough to assume her usual position.

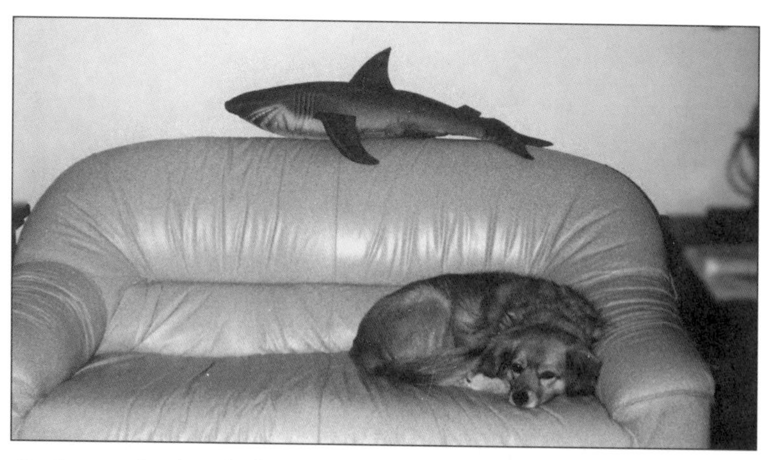

Perhaps she heeded primordial "whispers" that would have had survival value in the wild. Of course, it would take my husband to ask: Do natural predispositions give clues that could enhance our own well being?

"A Home for the Heart"

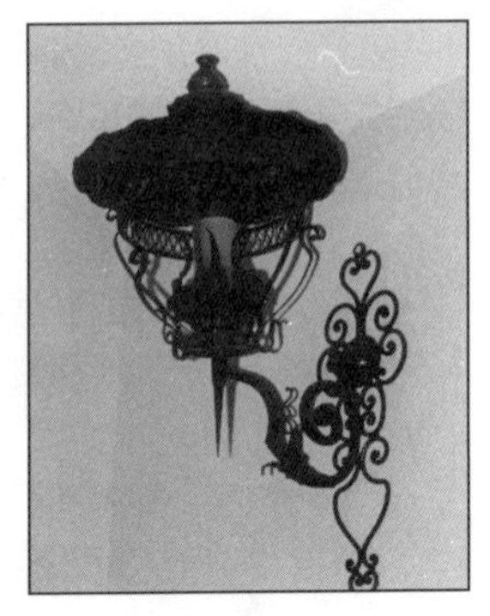

It wasn't long after moving to our country home that my ovarian cancer was diagnosed – turning my world upside down. This lovely country setting, though, was a stabilizing influence. Who knows but that the serenity, fresh air and nutrient-rich soil in which to garden didn't provide other health benefits. And we are more inclined to exercise as beautiful hiking trails abound. Even the outdoor Spanish lantern my husband treasures remains – indoors – something of a visual mantra.

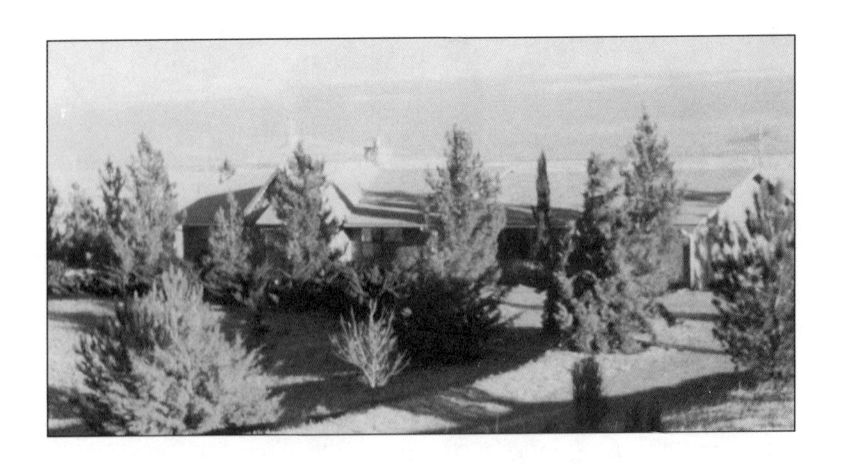

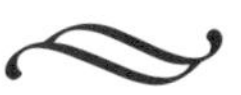

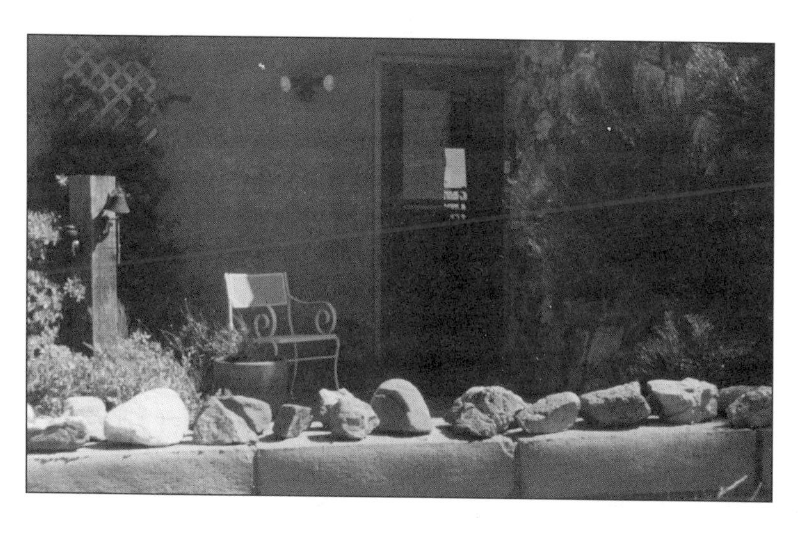

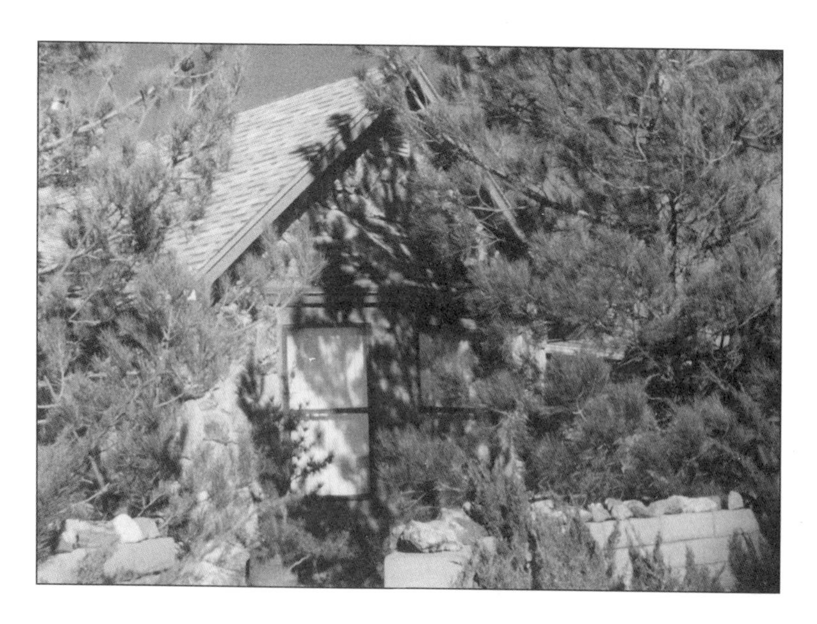

chapter sixteen

Learning to Live

The moment you realize the Grim Reaper has his eyes on you, your mind seemingly leaves the body in disbelief. Yet, a surrealistic awareness that it is you scheduled for extinction does emerge. The Reaper's shadow is now your companion.

Just how devastating this realization was is difficult to communicate but I can now understand why some victims simply bide time and wait. For one thing, the feeling that the inevitable can only happen to someone else is perennial. For another, accepting the word of the medical establishment that nothing else can be done is the line of least resistance and, indeed, besides discouraging one from seeking competitive treatment, it does fill cemeteries. And my experience in avoiding this murky fate taught me to be very proactive. Thus, my attitude meant everything.

To be sure, it's not just listening to pep talks, although that has its place. I address the potential victim this way: Do you have something to live for and are you willing to accommodate a considerable risk of failure if the answer is yes? Not only can I say with reasonable certainty that the phrase, "There is nothing more that can be done," is often an institutionalized lie, but going outside of the medical-pharmaceutical establishment is, typically, not that easy. No doubt, this is why those with solid reasons outside of simple self-preservation have a better chance because, for one, they are that much more motivated to overcome obstacles. And obstacles do predominate.

* * * *

The lack of time to effectively start an alternative treatment program very often results when a patient is only informed of his or her true prospects at the last possible minute. Not unlike most people, doctors do not like to admit defeat and often procrastinate. Some believe their own propaganda and assume no reason for urgency thinking no viable treatment options remain. Still others, no doubt, know the score but would feel their professionalism diminished by a patient breaking rank and successfully beating back his or her terminal illness. Thus, seriously ill cancer patients frequently overestimate their remaining time. It was making this mistake that nearly cost me my life, as mentioned earlier.

Charity work outlining my experiences by telephone, in person and, lately, through the internet has brought me in contact with over 300 cancer victims, many of whom were in their late terminal stages. In fact, I can only think of about 12 of this great number who early on investigated natural treatment possibilities to be used either as the sole modality or as an early complement to the conventional treatments they were receiving. One of the few is Marilyn Bollinger who I had mentioned followed a highly sensible course using both conventional and nontraditional treatment programs. Her recognition of "the silent killer" within, ovarian cancer, provided the time necessary to evaluate more benign treatment possibilities.

Fully realizing the average reader will already have – suspended by the clock's thinnest hair – a Damoclean sword overhead, I still plan to later detail Marilyn's unique case. It is hoped that such an approach will help convince more people to do some wide-ranging research even before any immediate need. In fact, this is a goal of the Cancer Control Society. Again, I must stress how extremely fortunate I was to have stumbled into, really, the single natural substance, shark cartilage, that proved effective in controlling my cancer. Had I been one of those for whom it didn't work, would John and I have had the considerable time necessary to research any number of other natural treatments not included in my regimen? A reality check suggests, probably not.

Our reality was that John especially sensed time was short and I started on the cartilage after only days of very intensive research. How much better off we would have been had we delved outside of the obvious much earlier and, therefore, had the time to truly explore all of our options is anyone's guess. John had noted at least eight critical junctures in which we might have turned the cartilage therapy aside. My improbable husband again could hardly resist calculating the probability of my ending up on the side of the cartilage, assuming a reasonable 50 percent chance of doing so at each of these junctures. His conclusion? Less than one percent! Needless to say, this all seemed so arcane and so like John that my first impulse was to praise his effort but otherwise suggest how crazy this sounds. But he did start me to thinking.

Looking back on July 12, 1994, the first day of the cartilage therapy, I remember how little we knew, how tentative our steps and how very, very fortunate we were. There is no doubt our intensive but truncated effort did pay off – but still, my being here to write these words did in some measure depend upon a fluke! According to my husband's statistical assumptions and obscure calculations, there was a 99-percent chance that this book would have never been started and he and "Pup" would have been left alone – and adrift. Interestingly, not only does John seem to somehow identify with our little dog, but as well, with the dog house. Perhaps my reaction to some of his conclusions is part of the reason.

To say that John is different is an understatement. Yet my intuition, indeed, does tell me I had the good fortune of listening to him at certain junctures. This is quite remarkable, actually, as on many occasions, I had solemnly vowed never to listen to him again.

* * * *

Yet I listened to John again as he described one technique he used to evaluate alternative cancer treatments. Interestingly, it is based on trends in the commercial markets.

John had noticed that the more successful stock market investors were those who increased their exposure when the prevailing winds were the most bearish. He noted also that few investors have the fortitude to use this contrariant approach because of the herd instinct. Going with the flow is so easy that it causes trends to continue beyond reasonable expectations and is especially evident in stock market bull runs ending in corrections or even spectacular crashes.

As to how the above could apply to evaluating nontoxic cancer treatments is perfectly clear to this husband of mine. You see, the huge pharmaceutical-medical cartel's deep money pockets help carry not only the FDA but the hub of government as well and, thus, largely directs the winds of influence. The sight, then, of millions of people lining up for chemotherapy or radiation with few considering competing nontoxic cancer treatments is to be expected. One must remember that the most effective cartels do perform at least some good and this is especially true of conventional health care which is often highly beneficial. Therefore, the fact that the American Medical Association and large pharmaceutical companies are some of the most generous contributors of cash in the political arena is cleverly obscured. The end health result, however, is that we Americans get less mileage from the health dollar and the war against cancer is still a hollow campaign.

This is not to imply that everyone in the alternative health field is concerned with the plight of the cancer victim. I can attest to some questionable apples in this barrel as well. The most objectionable are those humanoids who crawl out onto an alternative soapbox and fawn so as to minimize the cartel's disfavor. On the other hand, those who are angrily buffeted by the cartel's winds of influence may well be the ones with the most effective alternative cancer treatments – and this is the key to John's evaluation technique. That denounced by the all-wise cartel as somehow harboring "potential harm" or as the rendering works of "junk science" may be as good for you, as it was for me. But in uncovering this contrariant relationship, one seeming contradiction bothered John no end and, consequently, came under his increased scrutiny.

* * * *

John wondered why chiropractic was so nearly driven to extinction by the AMA that by 1987 the courts finally intervened. Although chiropractic theory posits the interference of nerve function as the cause of some disease states and radiography is used for spinal analysis, it otherwise seemed more a simple manual therapy, at least, in John's mind. Thus, it being reviled so savagely by the cartel apparently contradicted John's thesis as it didn't seem to compete directly with standard pharmaceutical medicine and, thus, should have been left alone in the same way massage therapies had been. As usual, John resorted to asking questions mainly of the people we knew. The process revealed extensive gaps in our own knowledge.

John had always viewed chiropractic as "fluff" and my impression of it was only moderately favorable. Someone told us that it was the only alternative therapy whose practitioners are licensed in all fifty states and we were immediately impressed not only by the high percentage of our friends and acquaintances who had undergone the treatment, but, also, by their positive impressions of it. "It's the only thing that keeps me going," one friend confided. Another said his chronic headaches were substantially reduced by one chiropractor's treatment (but not by others). Several seemed to use their chiropractic doctors for some primary care needs as the doctors were also knowledgeable about nutrition and natural remedies. In all, the responses were highly favorable and left us with the impression that chronic conditions unresponsive to conventional treatments were often alleviated by chiropractic manipulation.

John now knew why chiropractic had been subjected to such vicious attacks: it does, indeed, compete directly with conventional medicine essentially because it works! As expected, a fair number of negatives were heard: mainly, that the practitioners were sometimes inadequately skilled or "too far out." The fact that the chiropractors were well organized and had sufficient money to defend themselves in court was also apparent. But, alas, in cancer therapy for terminal cases, such is not always the case and promising nontoxic treatments have been all but stamped out. Interestingly, at different times I have used four of these, as already mentioned, for imune boosters: a variant of the Kelley diet featuring enzymes among other natural substances; Essiac herbal tea; a variation of the Hoxsey formula; and a safe intake of apricot kernels for vitamin B17.

The leading researcher of shark cartilage therapy, Dr. Lane, has been subjected to the usual attacks but many of these have been subtle. For example, I have read very short newspaper articles conspicuously relegated to the obscure pages which painted him as something of a maverick and bumpkin, without the conventional qualifications (an M.D. degree, of course) of a researcher. In one case, "a clinical trial" was set up whose protocol, among other limitations, allowed insufficient time and used an inferior brand of shark cartilage powder in an obvious move to suggest shark cartilage doesn't promote the control of cancer. Even the *National Geographic* magazine of June 1998 ran an article on the prospects of using certain potential tumor-inhibiting compounds derived from the common dogfish shark without mentioning Lane's name in its positive lead outlining previous research efforts. Of course, the snub was complete in the many recent reports I read of the two proteins, angiostatin and endostatin, curbing cancer in mice.

Not once in these reports was shark cartilage mentioned even though it appears to curb malignant growth in the same way by impeding a tumor's blood supply (antiangiogenesis). EntreMed is not the only company to profit by the prospect of turning the proteins into salable drugs as a number of companies less directly linked to this effort have also experienced very lucrative stock growth. <u>If</u> the expensive and lengthy development process is successfully completed and big money promises to be made, it will become available to save lives. What is here now is nontoxic but slower acting shark cartilage, thanks, chiefly, to Dr. Lane.

The cartel may have refrained from making noisy and openly vicious attacks on Dr. Lane because of the lessons learned in now 15 years of trying to suppress the work of Stanislaw Burzynski, M.D. In spending many millions of taxpayer dollars and causing the doctor's mostly terminal cancer patients much misery and expense, government bureaucrats failed to get very far. Perhaps they failed to understand that practicing members of the criminal justice system realize that they too must do some good apparent to the public to maintain their highly profitable closed system. And that is exactly what happened.

The beleaguered Burzynski had been hauled into so many grand jury sessions and court proceedings, it is actually difficult to keep count. Once in court, the worst that government prosecutors could do was to come up with one hung jury (in 1997, the subsequent jury found him not guilty on all counts). This bureaucratic nonsense no doubt killed some people desperate for Dr. Burzynski's nontoxic treatment but I doubt that the perpetrators would openly celebrate this outcome. Nor did government prosecutors relish their trumped-up charges being commonly thrown out by the judge. Furthermore, others had reason to fear bureaucratic meddling.

AID patients had a unique status because, though often terminal, they typically had many months or years to live and they were fully aware of the prejudice against them. As a result, they had the motivation and time to establish underground pharmacies and conduct clinical trials hoping to develop more effective treatment protocols – and, actually, they were quite successful. Although the AID patients felt that this prejudice stemmed from the disease's association with homosexuality, I believe <u>any</u> seriously ill patient who tries to survive using unconventional approaches may sometimes come under as much prejudice – some of it openly vicious. The offspring of one terminal patient I know of had to quietly obtain the shark cartilage requested by the parent because other family members objected. So government bureaucrats are not the only perpetrators of this form of discrimination. Hypocritically, though, all cancer patients, including those terminal, come under the "protection" of the Americans with Disabilities Act (ADA)!! One survey mentioned earlier suggested only six percent of the population had "a lot" of trust in government. Although this statistic has recently improved, there is little wonder why government bureaucrats are still held in such low regard stemming not only from this kind of hypocrisy but the IRS horror stories as well.

It is with good reason, then, that I maintain an ample supply of cartilage at all times for fear my supply could be cut off by government edict. We remember well that Dr. Burzynski's patients faced such a deadly quagmire. True, the nontoxic treatment was "antineoplastons," not shark cartilage. However, both Dr. Burzynski's medicine and the shark cartilage therapy championed by Dr. Lane, are outside of the conventional loop. When patients said they would die without the medicine, the bureaucratic attitude was, "So what?"

This book was not prepared because the subject is pleasant, but because surviving cancer victims like me need to make the true situation known. Had I been better prepared from the very beginning and had started my particular treatment regimen earlier, my story would have likely been shorter and happier. So let me give you an account of someone who was prepared and is now a dear friend. Her name is Marilyn Bollinger.

* * * *

Unfortunately, my case is a long litany of errors and virtually every cancer patient known to me had taken the same missteps I had. Consequently, my account is addressed in large measure to those in the final stages of the disease. Marilyn Bollinger, however, is one of the few who was up and ready when her ovarian cancer struck. In fact, it was an alternative massage therapist who discovered the suspicious abdominal lump on October 12, 1995 (the month and day John and I first met 47 years earlier!). Of course, this led to a medical verification and she started carboplatin therapy November 3 for her Stage III ovarian cancer.

Marilyn appeared to appreciate the mind/body connection and continued to read related materials especially on visualization while at the same time asking questions of those who might supply sound information including, appropriately, her oncologist (who is also mine).

On February 19, 1996, she underwent the laparoscopic removal of only the ovaries and omentum as the uterine tumors had been erased by the chemotherapy. Yet her condition was considered very serious and three days later taxol was added to the regimen. This conventional course of treatment ended April 25 of 1996 and henceforth she relied solely on nontoxic alternative approaches including exercise.

General and special stretching exercises were especially pursued and along with Yoga are now a significant part of her daily routine. In fact, riding her bicycle 10 or 15 miles is one of her less strenuous activities. A very active retiree, she frequently travels not only in this country but abroad to such diverse places as England and Sicily, to give but two examples.

On July 2, Marilyn became a part of my support group and I remember vividly how inquisitive she was concerning how I controlled my cancer. And just a month later she began a substantial maintenance regimen of the BeneFin shark cartilage powder. Not that she depended on the cartilage therapy alone! On July 5, she started homeopathic treatments; on September 11, psychotherapy; and a week later, shiatsu "acupressure" sessions.

In October, while still doing Yoga, she attended a Chi Gung workshop to learn more about energy healing and how to stimulate the body's internal and external energy circuits in order to promote healing.

In January of 1997, Marilyn started attending monthly workshops on alternative treatments for cancer. In February, she visited a hypnotherapist to better deal with fear and review self-hypnosis. At the end of April, she enrolled in a five-day seminar which featured the well-known medical doctors, Andrew Weil and Christiane Northrup, and emphasized alternative medicine as well as holistic avenues and self-healing. All the while, Marilyn still volunteered at The West Shop, a charitable outlet whose proceeds help needy women and children of Tucson.

In 1998, her CA-125 tumor marker crept up ever so slightly after she sharply lowered her cartilage intake to about 35 grams daily. Consequently, she increased the dosage to the former level of at least 65 grams daily and her marker moved downward and is currently below seven – well within the "safe" range of 35 or below.

Again and again, I have noticed remarkable differences among those who manage to successfully beat back their malignancies. Yet, almost all carefully make a decision and stick with it – regardless. In Marilyn's case, how was one to know which parts of her alternative regimen, if any, helped and which didn't? The mix was more complex because there may have been a synergistic feature involving some or even all of these parts. But this uncertainty didn't alter her comprehensive course.

In my case, only after a considerable time did it become crystal clear that it was the shark cartilage carrying the yeoman load in keeping me alive. It is beginning to appear the cartilage is doing the same in Marilyn's case. In fact, the oncologist seemed more than pleased over her marker remaining quite steady for about three years and very possibly responding to the cartilage.

To win, lose, or draw is part of life but being forearmed with knowledge garnered with an open mind does seem to improve one's prospects. If we lived in a more perfect world, preparing oneself for perilous contingencies might be easier. As it is, it takes a will to live. And there appears to be no best style in approaching the task.

For example, except for our both taking the cartilage, my approach was somewhat different from Marilyn's partly because my energy level is not nearly as high. All that traveling of itself would have worn me to a frazzle! Though styles may differ, we can learn from one another and form a coherent plan of action. And my experience tells me that the reader of this account will very likely be a late starter with no time to waste. It is with this in mind that I outline in the next chapter the nuts and bolts of my late start in the hope of making a real difference for you.

chapter seventeen

Nuts and Bolts and a Little More

Based on my experience, the reader here is likely to be in the final stages of terminal cancer. If my husband, hadn't sensed the urgency of my condition, I would have likely taken too much time in seeking out the cartilage therapy and thus died. And I now sense my death would have taken place at the end of 1995. Even now, what I am telling you is intensely unsettling as I saw no realistic hope and I could tell that John didn't either. Yet, at John's urging we plowed forward while shrouded in disbelief that this could have actually happened to me. At first, our actions were mechanical, doing something because the notion of doing nothing didn't really occur to us. Nevertheless, we quickly warmed up to the task as we came to realize that there was a world of possibilities out there – so many, in fact, we were forced to restrict our range of inquiry.

We focused our research only on those alternative treatments which had some solid data behind them primarily because John was afraid I had too little time left to do otherwise. The terminal reader also is likely to miscalculate the time remaining, a normal tendency that so nearly put me in an early grave. And by my not awakening sooner, a second error was almost inevitable: not taking enough of the cartilage powder at the very beginning. Simply put, I was not fully accustomed to the idea that a low-tech, natural treatment required not only more time to experience results but also a much greater daily intake than any harsh pharmaceutical counterpart would have (had it been available, of course). Instead of aiming to ingest one gram of the shark cartilage powder daily for every two pounds of body weight, I could have nearly doubled that, at least at the beginning. (When at 130 pounds, for example, I could have taken, say, 110 grams daily of the shark cartilage powder instead of the roughly 60 grams I might have been taking).

Although I did make sure my oral doses of the cartilage powder were mixed fresh each time in about eight ounces of a recommended liquid and taken on a completely empty stomach, I only learned belatedly that taking it a full hour before mealtime was extremely beneficial as indicated by my CA-125 tumor marker response. Perhaps the liquid of choice is cold water which goes fairly well with the orange flavored BeneFin brand shark cartilage powder. Orange, apple and grape are juices also recommended.

* * * *

There was one thing I did do right from the very beginning, it should be noted. I didn't immediately abandon the retention enemas which may have helped relieve my chemo-damaged digestive system. I had often taken two or three daily dosages of the regular shark cartilage powder this way, about 18 grams each mixed thoroughly in tepid water.

Because of the body's reflex, the enema at first proved difficult to retain for the recommended 30 minutes minimum. I experimented with both the conventional enema bag and the syringe but found their use awkward and wasteful of the mixture. Then it occurred to me that the ready-to-use clear plastic squeeze bottle the Fleet brand enema came in might do the trick. I emptied the bottle of its original liquid content and washed it thoroughly before carefully reassembling its four parts, including the flat one-way safety valve. And it proved convenient and far less wasteful. By thoroughly cleaning the squeeze bottle after each use, it lasted a month or more. I used a thick mat and lay on my right side as had been recommended by Dr. Lane for easier retention – yet stayed close to the toilet. Within a week or two, the procedure became so routine I was able to relax and listen to the radio. And in no time, I often retained the mixture indefinitely for increased absorption. At first, I cringed upon hearing of this time-consuming method but now look back upon the experience somewhat warmly – yet, short of longingly, to be sure.

* * * *

Because the cartilage therapy early on had doused my rheumatoid arthritis symptoms and just weeks later my abdominal cancer pain, I suspect I had a much easier time staying the course compared to those lacking such early indicators. Consequently, many late-stage cancer victims who start the therapy are talked out of it or respond to some part of the pharmaceutical cartel's well-oiled propaganda machine. Fortunately, those casting about to save themselves are typically above average in education and have, thereby, the wherewithal to do their own research and grasp the true situation but, unfortunately, often have neither the time remaining nor strength to do so adequately. From my experience, such a person needs a true companion (say, a spouse, relative or close friend) willing to help on a daily basis.

Remember, if just five percent more of the terminal cancer population could be rescued, the number saved yearly would be an astounding 25,000 lives! (Compare that with the relatively few lives saved yearly by vehicle air bags). It has been "leaked" that two of the first four Stage IV breast cancer patients participating in an FDA-approved East Coast clinical trial of BeneFin brand shark cartilage have had the progression of their terminal cancers halted and in one case, significantly reversed. And these were women with morbidly compromised immune systems! (See the June, 1998, issue of the *Alternatives* newsletter, Editor: Dr. David G. Williams, Mountain Home Publishing – for past issues call 800-718-8293, to subscribe, 800-219-8591.)

Unless a terminal cancer victim has at least some background knowledge of the health care industry, there is little hope of successfully sifting through the maze of conflicting information. Before me now is an article taken from the September 17, 1998 issue of a major Tucson newspaper, *The Arizona Daily Star*. Its title, "Journal of Medicine criticizes supplements" stretches across more than half of a page top in the paper's lead section even though only six reports of "severe illness" from supplements appeared in the then current New England Journal of Medicine, upon which the article was based! Reading this article made me all the more aware of just how much I have changed because of my cancer as it wasn't too many years ago I might have paid more heed to the size of the headline than the article's substance. But now I compare that tiny number, "six," with the millions who have suffered untoward reactions to pharmaceuticals, including those that had poisoned me!

According to the article, the suggestion was made that supplements should undergo the same rigorous testing that drug treatments do. And this, too, would have sounded reasonable to me, but now I know that this testing often costs many millions of dollars and would force almost all supplements off of the market. Why? No company is going to spend the money necessary to test, say, an age-old mushroom supplement for efficacy and safety if the plant can be grown in a person's garden and is not patentable.

This brought to mind my husband, John, who has a mild case of a chronic skin disease, psoriasis, whose scaly patches are now resistant to even the most potent prescription salves. Just recently, he learned of a natural combination consisting of mineral oil, some castor oil, and a very small amount of aloe vera gel, all of which can be purchased commercially. After thoroughly mixing these ingredients, he "painted" the affected areas with a brush and with periodic applications considerable healing took place with no developing "drug" resistance evident. Obviously, none of these natural ingredients had undergone the expensive testing that would be required under drug laws, (though in combination they did essentially act like drugs). Aloe vera gel, in particular, would be difficult to patent as the aloe vera plant can be cultivated and, in fact, is growing in my front yard!

We had heard of a government bureaucrat suggesting that if shark cartilage was "officially" proven to work, it would have to be considered a drug and taken off the market pending completion of the FDA approval process. Knowing what I know now, I have to ask, why wasn't broccoli taken off the market? However, I have learned, too, that absurdity does tend to follow absurdity, thus the reason for our stocking up... on shark cartilage, that is.

* * * *

Needless to say, I found it shocking that seriously ill cancer patients often face prejudice, principally by having treatment alternatives blocked. Curiously, I found those in need of organ transplants also face prejudice, but largely through apathy. And each case appears to revolve around money. It is a giant pharmaceutical cartel protecting its financial advantage on one hand and a system of organ procurement without much monetary incentive on the other. I had even learned patients facing this apathy weren't told, typically, that they could put their names on more than one transplant list to increase the chances of finding a suitable donor! (However, changes appear to have been made in organ procurement procedures in recent months.) For this reason the free-market dynamics found in alternative medicine doesn't bother me as much as the stagnation associated with a closed system. The cartel's central argument seems to be that people can't be trusted to make their own health choices and that a closed system is essential to keep everyone "safe." The classic one used by the world's dictators to justify their political existence is also seductively simple: people can't be trusted to govern themselves.

It goes without saying that freedom does bring about some absurdity. And it is my conclusion that it will always have a market. But if someone says he can divine the nature of your ills by contemplating your navel, you, as a free citizen, are likely to ask some probing questions or, simply, walk away. Still, an open mind is essential. Remember how improbable acupuncture sounded when it first came to this country? Similarly, it took the once alternative Heimlich maneuver about 10 years to become generally accepted. Since neither of these treatment forms competed directly with the cartel, each in its own way is today a valuable part of the standard medical arsenal.

I have found secondary media sources less mindful of the cartel's big money influence and, therefore, richer in alternative information. You might remember my mentioning that one mother saved her son using information given on a daytime talk show, hardly a prestigious source. In summary, I need to stress that without my having gained a realistic picture of how things really were I would not have been able to stick by my comprehensive program and, thus, save my life. The general picture provided by conventional sources, be they government bureaucracies, conventional charities or what have you, are incomplete and even misleading because they are each staffed with essentially the same kind of people. Interestingly, they often quote one another in news releases giving the impression there is only one true point of view.

* * * *

Sometimes, people seem to get wrapped up in my auxiliary efforts to boost my immune system thinking, perhaps, I was giving the cartilage therapy too much credit. And, indeed, I had been taking antioxidants and other substances, such as: B-complex vitamins, *Gingko biloba* and ginseng (Siberian); vitamin C and beta-carotene along with vitamin E coupled with the mineral, selenium; coenzyme Q10 (CoQ10); flaxseed oil (cold-pressed, organic); cat's claw *(Uncaria tomentosa)*; grape seed extract; soy products; garlic (cooked); *Lactobacillus acidophilus*; as well as maitake and other therapeutic mushrooms. These and other supplements mentioned previously (see Index), may have had an underlying benefit, but I did not discern that this auxiliary regimen had a major effect. In fact, this appeared to be the conclusion reached by my naturopathic physician.

It should be noted that I had been quite health conscious before contracting my cancer and had been on a some basic supplements very early on. True, this supplemental intake was expanded at the start of my shark cartilage therapy in July of 1994 but only modest modifications were made since, and, most convincingly, the unexpected positive therapeutic outcomes I did experience corresponded not only with the times I started and then restarted taking the shark cartilage but with its dosage changes as well.

Curiously, people haven't had that much regard for my auxiliary support program, even though my using self-hypnosis, visualization, and certain meditation techniques, coupled with gentle yoga exercises, had seemed a significant aid. And especially was this true of my support group attendance. Here, I listened to the cancer experiences of the other women and I felt less alone. And my gaining of information not otherwise readily available was another plus. For example, I discovered that another participant's CA-125 tumor marker of 2,000 equated in seriousness to my marker of 200 – at least, this was my impression. And since then, I talked to women with even much higher marker levels who were still functioning quite well. So now, I view any marker number using a more flexible perspective to gauge its significance.

While support groups no doubt vary in this regard, my group proved warm and mutually helpful. For many of the participants, the cancer group had become a second family. And I also view it this way. Only someone who has gone through the experience of fighting this terrible disease can fully understand the fearsome anxieties involved. Even though my naturopathic physician, especially, encouraged my attendance, the very positive experiences I had in the group, nevertheless, appeared to have had no real influence on the course of my malignancy. In fact, my highest tumor marker ever, 236.2, (which occurred nine months after going off the shark cartilage for surgeries) was registered some six months following my initial attendance of the support group in mid 1995. In hindsight, it was the downward but strangely "bouncy" behavior of the tumor markers which perhaps most clearly demonstrated that it was thc shark cartilage actually doing the major work.

All together, I have had at least 56 CA-125 tumor markers beginning with 118.9 registered June 9, 1992, just eight days before my hysterectomy which had led to my Stage III ovarian cancer diagnosis. If my memory is correct, another marker of 141 was gotten during this same period, but I cannot find it recorded anywhere.

On July 2, 1992, the marker was down to 42.1, apparently the result of the surgery and just above the "safe" range of 35 or less. On the same day, my long string of chemotherapy treatments began and the markers (17 of them) ranged between 7.2 and 15.2 until May 19, 1994 (nearly two years later) when a marker suddenly rose to 28.5, nearly three weeks before my very last chemotherapy treatment. On June 24, the marker registered an alarming 130.1 and six days later, Thursday, June 30, I was told the chemotherapy treatments had failed and that the gentler Tamoxifen and Megestrol would have to do because my imune system was now compromised. On July 12, I watchfully started on the shark cartilage therapy (soon, up to 60 grams daily) and that is when the tumor markers began behaving strangely as shown in the following sequence starting August 5, 1994, and ending March 8, 1995, (about seven months): 97.8 (down from 130.1) 113.0… 226.0 (increased cartilage dosage) 45.2… 50.9… 76.2… 68.1.

On March 25, 1995, my "benign" brain tumor was surgically removed and just days earlier I had ceased taking the shark cartilage and for more than nine months remained off of it as recommended because of a series of surgeries that became necessary. During this time I had substituted the recommended dosage of at least nine grams daily of bovine cartilage for the antiangeogenic shark cartilage powder and I had even been taken off of the hormonal therapy, Tamoxifen and Megestrol, by my oncologist because, as he suggested, something else was at work here which was more effective. And for a while, things were looking up because the markers continued to go down – for a time. Note how smoothly the tumor markers behaved when I was <u>not</u> taking the shark cartilage as demonstrated in the following sequence beginning April 11, 1995, and ending January 2, 1996, (almost nine months): 25.1 (hormonal therapy stopped) 23.6… 13.1… 11.3… 27.5… 145.7… 188.5… 236.2.

It should be noted that John had talked to a West Coast naturopathic cartilage researcher who suggested the initial downturn may not have been caused by a lingering effect of the previous shark cartilage therapy but by the excision of the brain tumor itself which may have been malignant, though undetected as such. Be that as it may, I returned to taking about 65 gram daily of the BeneFin shark cartilage powder January 9, 1996 while also remaining on the bovine cartilage (for another nine months). While the following sequence involved some changes in the shark cartilage dosages, the "bouncy" behavior of the tumor markers was unmistakable and, therefore, only the major dosage changes are noted. The sequence begins with the March 7, 1996 marker and ends with that of July 28, 1998 (ranging well over two years): 95.6 (down from 236.2 of nine weeks earlier!) 70.5… 46.1… 49.9… 72.9 (greatly increased dosage) 37.2… 12.4 (decreased dosage) 35.5… 27.1… 30.6… 22.0… 23.0… 35.9… 35.7… 27.1 (made sure at least 45 minutes passed between dosage and meal) 18.7… 2.5… 5.0. (A major symptom of the cancer's return, the chronic morning diarrhea which began December 14, 1995, also disappeared early in this period, April 12, 1996 to be exact.)

Virtually all health professionals familiar with the details of my case concluded the shark cartilage obviously helped control my cancer. In fact, the somewhat odd tasting powder now seemed to be working better than it ever had. Along the way, I had learned some valuable lessons, even from this ever watchful husband of mine.

John's insistence that everything be carefully checked and measured now makes sense to me. And the way he double checks my shark cartilage dosage levels might best be given in the form of an actual example: For now, I want to maintain a daily dosage level of between 65 and 70 grams. By dividing 454 (the number of grams in a pound of cartilage powder) by 67.5 (the midpoint between 65 and 70) he obtained the quotient of 6.7 which represents the approximate number of days and a fraction a pound container of cartilage powder should last. Thus, based on this calculation alone, he can estimate, upon my finishing a container, just how close I came to my daily target. But as you might guess, knowing John's peculiar ways, this was not the end of it... as you will see.

To meet this daily target, I ingest three well-rounded scoops of the BeneFin powder (mixed thoroughly in a glass of cold water and taken on an empty stomach) three times a day, the three mixtures taken as far apart during the day as feasible. (A scoop comes in the BeneFin container and equals a little less than a tablespoon). Since I use a total of nine rounded scoops per day, John divided the day, correspondingly, into nine parts. Consequently, the number, 1 (one day) was divided by the 9 which equals, .111 – hence, each scoop represents a hair above 11 percent of a day's total intake. Now to try and illustrate how he uses all this: On September 4, I emptied a 454 gram cartilage container after the fourth full scoop equaling, .44 (4 x .11) of the day's total intake. The new bottle ran out after 2-1/3 scoops for September 12 equaling approximately .26 (2 x .11 = .22 + .04 = .26) of this day's total.

Since the container lasted just under eight days, he subtracted .26 from .44, which indicated that I was shy .18 of the full eighth day. Thus, he determined the container lasted 7.82 days. But during this period I had taken 40 capsules (30 grams) of the cartilage from another bottle to take while away from home, so instead of ingesting just 454 grams, I had taken 30 grams more. Consequently, in this case he divided 484 (not 454) by the 7.82 which equals, 61.9, the average amount of cartilage in grams taken daily, somewhat short of the 65 to 70 grams I had intended to ingest. Again, all this makes perfect sense to John and as was his wont he told me about the deficit.

* * * *

What I hope to see in my remaining lifetime is a change toward medical freedom which would allow natural, nontoxic approaches to be integrated with standard medical practices which in its own right, it should be emphasized, is largely beneficial. In fact, even conventional cancer treatments often help, something I have witnessed first hand. Thus, medical freedom is not likely to lead to the wholesale displacement of the pharmaceutical industry as some might fear. John was recently diagnosed with skin cancer (thankfully, not melanoma) and has already undergone minor surgery for it, which for this type of cancer is very effective. Yet, he is forced to go "underground" to see what specific alternative treatments might also help. In a truly free country this impediment to alternative information designed to favor the wealthy pharmaceutical cartel would not exist.

Nevertheless, with so many people seeking out alternative information and treatments, I sense change is in the air. But change is never easy. The veterinary profession has been known for treating animals humanely by using treatment options that work, whether they be pharmaceutical or natural. But just recently I read of a licensed chiropractor facing a possible five-year prison sentence for successfully treating dogs for a type of chronic pain apparently unresponsive to normal veterinary therapy! For sure, the road to change will likely be strewn with some unbelievable obstacles. The most unbelievable I have encountered so far, though, is the suggestion by the one medical doctor that a terminal cancer patient should not risk trying "unproven" alternatives.

* * * *

It is hard to believe that my ovarian cancer, while hardly in the background, is far from consuming my thoughts as it once did. In fact, I realized a few days ago that I had actually hit my old stride by trying to reform John of some of his bad habits. Although a half-century of effort had produced so little, just returning to this familiar endeavor really meant a lot: it was like walking through the threshold again. However, as before, I don't think John gave it that much notice. Perhaps it is just as well that some things never change.

chapter eighteen

An Afterword and Then Some

The ground swell of interest in alternative health seemed all the more apparent in recent months. And our many contacts about this book also revealed the grass-roots nature of this emergence – made all the more spectacular, perhaps, by some lack of formal leadership being evident. Our efforts must have been joined by those of millions of people who also sought to improve their health – "naturally," to use the term now repeated in expensive TV ads. And along with John and me, these millions had actually been leading the way, at least generally. And according to John, even our little dog is to be counted.

My husband's suggestion that nine-year-old "Coco" was somehow a part of this ground swell strained my belief but I hoped his explanation would not sound too crazy. You may remember that our dog's hind legs were "locked up" by osteoarthritis and she was treated with Chondroitin-Glucosamine (coupled, initially, with hefty amounts of pure bovine cartilage) which relieved the symptoms within days. When I tried cutting back the dosage level once again as suggested by the veterinarian, her arthritis symptoms reappeared and I had to increase the daily dosage some. Immediately, the symptoms again faded and then disappeared. This again greatly impressed John because a placebo effect could not have been a factor. Also, it should be noted, more dietary protein may have helped revive her. Then it happened!

When young, our dog balanced herself on her hind legs and wobbled about upright in order to see over a knoll or similar obstruction. By counting slowly, John had actually timed this feat for three or four seconds. Yet, many years later, her arthritic hind legs simply collapsed. Just the other night, though, up she went to peer over a spindly bush and, behold, she was fully upright wobbling about for at least three seconds and John appeared dumbfounded. "Of all the 'proofs' that there is something to this stuff, this is it," said he who must analyze everything.

I reminded him that he had recently started increasing his own protein consumption and not only did he experience weight reduction but increased energy as well. I also reminded him how his ingestion of cartilage had all but eliminated his arthritis. Then I asked him if the totality of our own positive experiences with natural remedies didn't carry even greater scientific weight? And his answer was no. OK, John, whatever.

* * * *

Actually, my tumor marker inched up one point to 6.0 by October 20, 1998, and then up to a 30.0 by March 3, 1999, a possible placebo effect not withstanding. My feelings were so positive that despite the extended interval between blood draws, I didn't call ahead for this latest marker before my next physical exam the 18th of March. Thus, when my oncologist informed me of it, I was surprised. Perhaps because of my reaction, the examination was intense. But happily, he found "nothing suspicious." Then he told me to go to the waiting room and get John and that he'd return in a few minutes. When I told John of the rise, he said that he had expected it. While we awaited the doctor, John reminded me that my shark cartilage experience had shown that a deep marker decline was always linked to a subsequent rise. It was then he told me to request having a CA-125 tumor marker assay every two months again because this four-month interval was too long and had upset his record keeping. "Who knows but that the marker had been higher and is now on its way down," he said. Regardless, I sensed dosage changes were in the offing.

When my oncologist returned, he sat back with a mildly concerned expression and turned to John. It was clear to both of us that he was there to listen and, of course, John responded.

Although I observed such episodes on many different occasions, I still found this session fascinating because it was John who was again ardently discussing health information and John's earlier indifference toward such matters is still a vivid memory. Yet, John sounded authoritative when he recounted for my oncologist the conversation he had with "an East Coast researcher" and how it was emphasized that shark cartilage therapy is not a cure but a holding action and that there was but little doubt that my ovarian cancer was still with me. "In fact," John said, "it appears that some Japanese researchers in particular are emphasizing cancer control over a cure." He went on to explain that the dosage requirements, especially for well-fed Americans, are higher than once believed and, significantly, when I am on the high dosages of shark cartilage my tumor markers behave rather erratically.

But my doctor said a tumor marker moving up to 30 or so is not considered serious unless accompanied by symptoms and in a case like mine – even without the involvement of shark cartilage – no alarm bells go off and "we would do nothing but continue monitoring." My using a new lab was also discussed as a possible factor. Then, strangely, my doctor appeared to have doubts about the bouncy marker behavior being related to my shark cartilage regimen. "When it is all plotted out," John replied, "this connection is clearly evident." My doctor then told us that my marker assay should be done once every two months and that I should now see him in six rather than eight months. Interestingly, my going back on a two-month tumor marker schedule was taken care of without my having to ask.

* * * *

From the beginning, John opposed the recent changes I had made in my daily dosage schedule. I had been taking my last daily dose of shark cartilage at bedtime and while this procedure did spread out the daily intake more, it also left me hungry and sleeping less well. So I had started taking it an hour earlier to allow for a bedtime snack. As you may remember, John was likewise unhappy when I stopped taking a dose in the middle of the night. Besides all this, my daily intake recently drifted downward slightly to about 65 grams yet John hadn't said that much about it. In fact, relaxed discussion had now become his primary avenue of persuasion and, obviously, it had little effect as I had drawn my own conclusions.

Yet, his softer approach had its rewards. For example, when we took my not-so-old sewing machine in for service, John spotted a highly computerized model on sale (John loves a good sale) and encouraged me to simply trade in my old machine and buy it. I can't say his old chauvinism didn't come to mind, but it didn't matter. Such largess is hardly an everyday event and I immediately concurred. After all, it is John who is the tight spender – and my new machine *is* lovely. But now it was the evening of March 18 and after dinner I told him, " I think we need to relax and discuss a new strategy."

* * * *

We sat at the kitchen table. John folded his hands in thoughtful repose and suggested a very early cartilage dose might not disturb my sleep. The idea of taking just two rounded scoops (13 grams or so) about four AM, when my deep sleep ended, took hold. Increasing the three waking dosages from three to four rounded scoops each was also decided on for a daily intake of 14 rounded scoops (14 x 6.67 = 93 plus grams). Thus, a pound container (454 grams) of cartilage powder would last just under five days. (A level scoop equals about six grams; a rounded scoop – not heaping – adds about two-thirds of a gram more for a total of about 6.67 grams. The white scoop itself, remember, comes with each container of the BeneFin brand of shark cartilage powder). I also decided to re-establish my former intake levels of the antioxidants, flaxseed oil, and, especially, the digestive enzymes cut back slightly in response to all the good news, particularly the 2.5 tumor marker of mid 1998.

John thought "the nighttime caper" (as he called the early morning cartilage schedule) was by far the most important change as it helped ensure systemic saturation around the clock. But still, these other steps seemed to brighten his mood as did my decision to follow the two-week intensive dosing procedure for the MGN-3 (Lane Labs-USA, Inc., distributor) that John and I had thought superfluous when first incorporating this clinically tested substance about six months ago. Obviously, my own immune system hasn't been adequate in fighting cancer and there is considerable evidence that this easy-to-take natural compound may provide a life saving immunologic boost. For example, the results of one small clinical study showed that six (55 percent) of 11 cancer patients using MGN-3 experienced full remission and an additional three (27 percent) had partial benefit (*International Journal of Immunotherapy* 95; XI (I):23-28). Significantly, it may help to control cancers for which shark cartilage seems less effective, e.g., lymphoma, leukemia, and lung cancer. (Again, see the June, 1998, issue of the *Alternatives* newsletter, Editor: Dr. David G. Williams – refer to page 199.)

* * * *

Speaking of effectiveness, I am sometimes asked why I didn't first consider going outside this country to a cancer clinic in Mexico or even one in Germany or Switzerland. Lacking firsthand experience, I chose to limit discussion of these clinics even though several are located just across the California border in Mexico. Although their treatments may differ, the clinics seem to single-mindedly focus on being successful partly because word-of-mouth is such a powerful advertising medium.

Increased dependence, though, may be an unintended consequence of such a "packaged" regimen and, contrastingly, the successful terminal patients I have observed not only tend to be well educated, but also tend to take charge of their health and have a liberal sprinkling of independence. John and I may fit this description since we moved against my disease essentially on our own. This is not to say, however, such clinics are not worthy of investigation as some of their success stories are compelling. In fact, I am now looking at a fairly recent advertisement of the Center for Integrative Medicine at CHIPSA (Hositalario Internacional Pacifico, SA) which has a comprehensive immunotherapy program developed by a highly respected medical doctor – recently deceased – by the name of Josef M. Issels. While the ad reports an 87 percent long-term remission rate for those patients treated early, the rate reported for those patients who had exhausted all standard treatments was just under 20 percent. Obviously, even a highly respected clinic cannot make up for procrastination – at least not fully. Remember, there are quite a number of clinics in Mexico worthy of investigation and the Cancer Control Society of California is a good source of pertinent information (see the CCS listing under Useful Sources of Information).

One recent event again reminded me of our own procastination in investigating nonconventional options. Chemotherapy, remember, had damaged my left leg blood vessels so severely that I now face a lifetime of taking an anticoagulant or blood thinner. Just a few weeks ago, my "protime" tripled unexpectedly to well beyond the "safe" range and I faced the very real prospect of fatal bleeding. The thought still haunts me that had I been an informed consumer much earlier, it might have reduced the need for the damaging chemotherapy in the first place – the effects, of which, will now last my lifetime.

* * * *

The night before last Halloween, Tom Brokaw of NBC News announced that the seriously flawed clinical study I had briefly mentioned earlier had somehow determined that shark cartilage did not work to control cancer! Not mentioned in this NBC News report (apparently taken from an AP wire), the clinical trial initially consisted of 60 terminal cancer patients **and, reportedly, only a fraction of that number (15) actually completed the minimum of 12 weeks cartilage ingestion.** Apparently, none of the 60 late-stage cancer patients experienced tumor reduction, only temporary stabilization. And no wonder! For one thing, it takes shark cartilage therapy longer than 12 weeks for most people to have such a positive effect. You might remember, it took 20 weeks before my doctors and I had the first solid indication that the cartilage was working for me (my tumor marker dropped from 226 to 45).

Furthermore, the generic shark cartilage used was shown in Dr. Lott's study (see Chapter Four) to be much less antiangiogenic compared to the delicately processed BeneFin brand now being used in a FDA-sanctioned trial which had already shown a positive result. Reportedly, of four late-stage breast cancer patients who completed 20 weeks of therapy using BeneFin, one had a 25 percent reduction in a neck metastasis plus a complete response in a lung metastasis. Another subject had her disease stabilized. This study took place at a well known Medical Center in New Jersey. Numerous other studies, including a study by one of the NCI-trained cartilage researchers who assisted "60 Minutes," also contradict the negative results of this obviously flawed study which, nonetheless, was the one that made the headlines.

"Media short on credibility? Newspeople think so, too." This newspaper headline appeared in the lead section of the Arizona Daily Star on March 31, 1999. A poll of professional journalists by the Pew Research Center found that a whopping 69 percent agreed that the distinction between reporting and commentary has seriously eroded and a troubling 40 percent agreed that news reports are now full of factual errors and sloppy reporting!! So, who do you believe?

Not scientists, necessarily. Here, too, instances of questionable behavior proliferate. Most people realize, for example, that "expert witnesses" – often scientists – advertise in legal journals and are commonly available for a price to testify in a court of law to anything desired by a wealthy prosecutor or defense attorney. But fewer may be cognizant of the historical role of some scientists in promoting and otherwise providing the means for political despotism. In a word, they cannot always be regarded as simon-pure oracles of truth. But there was one report on "60 Minutes" that somehow had a refreshing ring to it.

This CBS News magazine on Easter Sunday, April 4, 1999, featured a report of a new antiangiogenic drug called, SU 5416. The UCLA Cancer Center for many months had conducted a clinical trial administering the drug to 63 terminal cancer patients and, encouragingly, 17 of the 63 subjects (27 percent) experienced either tumor shrinkage or tumor stabilization!

Several of the patients suffered blood clots and two of them died from heart attacks, but a hospital investigation suggested that the SU 5416 may not have been responsible. And one patient who had been doing remarkably well, died after his malignancy unexpectedly flared up. Yet, this angiogenesis inhibitor may ultimately play a valuable role.

It was a "60 Minutes" program in February of 1993, remember, that reported on another angiogenesis inhibitor, shark cartilage. Of the 29 terminal patients in that Cuban study, 14 survived and there were no blood clots or heart attacks observed. Furthermore, x-rays of some excised tumors showed clear evidence of a distinctive type of inner tumor disintegration coupled with encapsulation. But the National Cancer Institute showed overwhelming reluctance to follow up on that study. But, now, what a difference money makes!

In the 1999 program, there was considerable discussion about how much money was to be made if SU 5416 or a similar drug proves marketable. And, lo, the National Cancer Institute is funding the next phase of testing for SU 5416, according to the producers of the program. Newly diagnosed patients, it seems, will receive this drug along with chemo and/or radiation (perhaps allowing for a three-way profit potential). Prophetically, there was some discussion that all this research may **not** result in a cure for cancer after all, but may only help to manage it as a chronic disease! This is something many holistic researchers have been saying for years.

Five days following this "60 Minutes" program, NBC's "Dateline" featured a segment about a highly respected cancer doctor and surgeon who himself had colon cancer for which all conventional treatments, including surgery, failed. At his wife's urging he ventured into the alternative field, first doing meditation exercises which, because they seemed helpful, encouraged him to investigate further. Using the internet, he responded to the advice given by a highly respected Chinese herbalist by administering the recommended herbs initially to laboratory mice implanted with some of his malignant tissue. Incredibly, these implanted tumors stopped growing and shrank – as did his own remaining tumors sometime later after *he* ingested the herbs!!

According to the report, this highly placed medical doctor and five-year cancer survivor is now lecturing world-wide for more openness toward alternatives in the treatment of cancer and other diseases. And, significantly, not only did this NBC "Dateline" report seem essentially objective, but apparently this fine doctor hadn't been threatened with jail or otherwise harassed for exercising his First Amendment right! Correspondingly, in my informative role on a telephone network, I now find more medical people making inquiries about my experience. Indeed, the political climate does seem to be changing... but, sadly, only after the passage of so many years!

For decades, as mentioned earlier, the suppliers of nutritional supplements were not allowed to include critical information on their product labels. But the political influence of the large pharmaceutical companies entering the natural health field may have played a part in at least one positive outcome. According to the July, 1999, *Special Supplement* to the Julian Whitaker, M.D., *Health & Healing* newsletter, the Circuit Court of Appeals finally ruled this FDA imposed censorship violated the Constitution's guarantee of free speech – this after billions of containers of supplements were sold **with absolutely no label information** explaining what the product is supposed to do!

Another positive but personal outcome should be noted. Dear hubby was right about the nominal rise of my previous CA-125 tumor marker as the numbers tended downward again. The marker of May 4, 1999, was 24 (down from 30), and the marker of June 29 was 27, again, well within the "normal" range of 35 or less. We were forced to change to another HMO and thus to a new lab, and we strongly suspect that this lab's assay procedure may have played a part in determining these last three markers. Apparently different labs use different procedures.

My dear husband just voiced his concern that my chronicle might keep on going and going... perhaps for years. I protested that I still had important matters to discuss about the new millennium. Then there was silence. More than once he had suggested that all the talking I do in the GYN support group and on the telephone network just seems to continue without letup. So after a few minutes of quiet reflection, the realization struck me... the very least I could do is show him I can stop writing.

Useful Sources of Information

BOOKS

The following listing is tiny compared to the number of alternative health books available. Simply put, these few books were chosen from a sizable number of books which had been read or consulted. While a large book store is likely to feature a fine selection of alternative titles, a smaller health-oriented establishment may also carry a viable selection. Regardless, in this age of electronic communication, a fine old standby, the book, should not be forgotten.

Atkins, Robert C., M.D. *Dr. Atkins' Vita-Nutrient Solution.* New York, NY: Simon & Schuster, 1998.

Balch, James F., M.D., and Phyllis A. Balch, C.N.C. *Prescription for Nutritional Healing.* Second edition. Garden City Park, NY: Avery Publishing Group, 1997.

Bognar, David. *Cancer: Increasing Your Odds for Survival.* Alameda, CA: Hunter House, 1998.

Diamond, W. John, M.D., and W. Lee Cowden, M.D., with Burton Goldberg. *An Alternatiive Medicine Definitive Guide to Cancer.* Tiburon, CA: Future Medicine Publishing, 1997.

Lane, I. William, Ph.D., and Linda Comac. *Sharks Don't Get Cancer.* Updated edition. Garden City Park, NY: Avery Publishing Group, 1993.

Lane, I. William, Ph.D., and Linda Comac. *Sharks Still Don't Get Cancer.* Garden City Park, NY: Avery Publishing Group, 1996.

Lane, I. William, Ph.D., and Linda Comac. *The Skin Cancer Answer.* Garden City Park, NY: Avery Publishing Group, 1999.

Moss, Ralph W., Ph.D., *The Cancer Industry.* New updated edition. Brooklyn, NY: Equinox Press, 1996.

Moss, Ralph W., Ph.D., *Questioning Chemotherapy.* Brooklyn, NY: Equinox Press, 1995.

Quillin, Patrick, Ph.D.,R.D., with Noreen Quillin. *Beating Cancer With Nutrition.* Tulsa, OK: Nutrition Times Press, Inc., 1994.

Other Sources

An excellent 20-minute 1996 video tape, "Shark Cartilage: A Promise Kept," is available from: **Cartilage Consultants, Inc.**, of Short Hills, New Jersey. Phone: 800-742-7534. (Each of the three books by Lane and Comac listed here may also be ordered.)

Video tapes of the 1998 four-hour public television documentary, "Cancer: Increasing Your Odds for Survival," hosted by Walter Cronkite is also available for purchase from **New Way Productions** of Manchester, Connecticut. Phone toll-free: 888-307-4482. (The book of the same title by Bognar listed above is based on this public television special.)

One nonprofit organization in Otho, Iowa, **People Against Cancer,** is a public interest group which is equipped to provide valuable alternative information and offers a low-cost advisory service based on a cancer patient's specific medical history. Phone: 515-972-4444.

Another nonprofit organization in Los Angeles, California, the **Cancer Control Society**, holds an annual convention and conference over the three-day Labor Day weekend. The cost is nominal and the public is invited. It is a splendid opportunity to hear and meet alternative researchers and health care practitioners from around the country and beyond. Phone: 323-663-7801.

Ralph W. Moss, Ph.D., author of several ground-breaking books, two of which are listed here, offers his own alternative advisory service at low cost again based on a cancer patient's specific medical history. Phone: 718-636-4433 (Brooklyn, New York).

Cartilage Consultants, Inc., offers an excellent and free (save for the call to Southington, Connecticut) counseling service on the proper use of the BeneFin brand of shark cartilage and MGN-3. The counselor, **Marian Murphy** – a terminal cancer survivor herself – can also put you in touch with doctors familiar with the therapeutic potential of cartilage. Phone: 860-628-6061. This office is open for calls Monday through Thursday, 10 AM to 4 PM.

Another number to call for information is 800-510-2010 (CompassioNet, retailer of Lane Labs products including BeneFin brand shark cartilage and MGN-3).

The Center for Natural Medicine of Portland, Oregon has naturopathic, chiropractic and medical doctors, as well as specialists in acupuncture and massage. **Martin Milner, N.D.**, who heads this progressive clinic, is also a researcher and author and is familiar with shark cartilage therapy. Phone: 503-232-1100; Fax: 503-232-7751; E-mail: drmilner@hotmail.com

Dr. Milner is the author of a two-hour audiocassette (includes program and accompanying resource guide), "Prevent, Reverse and Survive Cancer" which may be ordered by calling 800-981-7157.

Klabin Marketing/Longevity Science of New York, NY is another fine source of nutritional supplements including the BeneFin brand of shark cartilage, all at discounted prices. Noted for their knowledgeable customer service, they carry the entire supplement line recommended by **Dr. Dante Ruccio** (see Introduction). Copies of this book may also be ordered here. Phone: 800-933-9440 or 212-877-3632. Fax: 212-580-4329.

The authors of this book, **Kay and John Bevan**, may be reached at their e-mail address: char@dakotacom.net Fax or phone: 520-455-5331.

An informed health care consumer
is an empowered one!

INDEX

A

B

C

Unfortunately, no government agency tabulates the outcome of various efforts to control cancer by alternative approaches, and thus, related information is scant. Additionally, many avoid even the thought of cancer until it finally erupts and affects them personally. This is why the reader is encouraged to share this book with others.

For ordering information, including quantity purchases, please note the following:

CHARHILL VOICE, LLC
Kay and John Bevan
PO Box 344
Sonoita, Arizona 85637-0344

E-mail: char@dakotacom.net
Fax or Phone: (520) 455-5331

NOTES:

NOTES:

NOTES: